A SAMPLING OF NATURE'S CURES

DID YOU KNOW . . . ?

- *Rosemary* can give you relief from a headache
- *Chamomile* will not only help you sleep, but is also an effective remedy for stress and upset stomach
- *Peppermint* and *Elderflower* will chase away the chills
- *Licorice* has been shown to cleanse the blood and clear the complexion
- *Ginger Root* is used all over the world for a variety of ailments
- *Fennel* was given to Olympic athletes by the Greeks for strength
- *Herb teas* are a safe alternative to drugs for nervous tension

Look to Nature *first*, and experience the "feel-good" miracle of maintaining a harmonious body balance that can mean a lifetime of health and well-being

D1210974

A
HANDBOOK
OF
NATURAL
FOLK REMEDIES

ELENA OUMANO, Ph.D.

AVON BOOKS ◆ NEW YORK

AVON BOOKS
A division of
The Hearst Corporation
1350 Avenue of the Americas
New York, New York 10019

Copyright © 1997 by Elena Oumano, Ph.D.
Published by arrangement with the author
Visit our website at **http://AvonBooks.com**
Library of Congress Catalog Card Number: 96-96920
ISBN: 0-380-78448-3

First Avon Books Printing: March 1997

AVON TRADEMARK REG. U.S. PAT. OFF. AND IN OTHER COUNTRIES, MARCA REGISTRADA, HECHO EN U.S.A.

Printed in the U.S.A.

RA   10 9 8 7 6 5 4 3 2 1

The advice and remedies offered in this book are not intended to be a substitute for the advice and counsel of your personal physician. Should you desire additional information or if you have any questions as to how this information pertains to you in particular, consult your doctor, nurse, pharmacist, or other health care provider.

Contents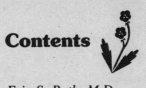

Contents

A
HANDBOOK
OF
NATURAL
FOLK REMEDIES

Foreword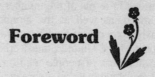

Technological advances in conventional medicine's diagnostic techniques and treatments have progressively increased Americans' average life expectancy without necessarily increasing the number of *quality* life years. People in this country live longer but often with more disease and much discomfort.

The widespread use of technology in medicine is wonderful, of course, but it has also created a complacency on the part of many practitioners in terms of making a diagnosis. Instead of relying on information gathered from observation and touch, there is a tendency to rely on the results of various sophisticated tests. In fact, these test results sometimes complicate a case by revealing findings which may not be relevant to the patient's complaints. This over-reliance on medical technology is also strongly influenced by a fear of litigation on the part of some practitioners. In addition, too many practitioners overuse medications. An example is the recent re-emergence of numerous infectious diseases which had been previously well controlled. This is the direct result of over-prescriptions of antibiotics, which, in turn, created resistant strains of bacteria. Far too few doctors focus their attention on natural alternative remedies that bolster the body's own immune powers, as well as preventative health care measures. Nor do they educate their patients as to how they can participate in their own health care.

Another problem today is the many choices of medical plans and types of coverage, which can prove very confusing to the average person. One has to become more aware of insurance regulations in terms of the number of visits and the type of tests allowed, as well as the number of treatments covered. Obviously, expense of health coverage must be considered. One aspect of the United States' crisis in health care is the increasing numbers of people who have no health insurance at all. They crowd hospital emergency rooms, thereby escalating health care costs dramatically, or they receive no health care at all. Even those fortunate enough to have health care insurance are not spared.

Due to the regulations of HMOs, coverage may end up being inadequate for *reasonable* treatment of a given condition, resulting in out-of-pocket expenses. There may not even be significant improvement following a course of treatment. A good example of this problem is a person who has suffered a traumatic injury which has resulted in musculoskeletal pain. All too often, this person receives improper treatment during the acute period. Once his condition becomes chronic, it usually becomes very difficult or impossible to correct the condition completely. As a result, when proper treatment is finally administered, it may be necessary to continue those treatments indefinitely in order for that person to carry on daily activities. I've encountered many situations where a successful treatment program was interrupted by limitations of health coverage. If the patient had been educated as to his options, he or she may have sought proper treatments during the acute period and would have been able to cure the condition. Very often, the proper treatment is not a conventional one.

This situation can become very frustrating and, as a result, more and more people are seeking out alternative medical treatments.

In my own practice, I have encountered a large set of patients who are very frustrated by the ineffectiveness of orthodox medical treatments and its over-reliance on prescription medications. I have found a willingness to try alternative forms of treatment such as acupuncture, homeopathy, herbs, and various hands-on treatments. The tremendous surge in the popularity of herbal and folk remedies we see today is a direct result of widespread disillusionment with conventional medicine.

Why bother with time-consuming, messy home remedies when you can pop a mass-produced wonder pill? Because all too often, prescription drugs patch up symptoms without addressing the causes. More significant, no one is sure of the long-term effects of these drugs. Few doctors would disagree that there is no safe drug.

Many drugs are made by synthesizing a particular property of an herb because that property is deemed to be the medicinal factor. For that reason, some medical experts argue that prescription drugs are actually more powerful and effective. But proponents of natural medicine have long argued that isolating and synthesizing a single ingredient of an herb removes it from an entire complex. Working synergistically and in harmony, the complex—rather than the single ingredient—might well be the actual source of the herb's healing properties. Isolating that single aspect might also remove elements that counteract any potential harm to the user.

It is my opinion that these forms of treatment are often more effective, less harmful, and less expensive. The problem for the average person then becomes trying to figure out which of these alternative treatments is appropriate for him.

The Handbook of Natural Folk Remedies pulls together solid and reliable information on remedies that have proven over centuries to be effective for a variety of ailments. It also integrates modern medical knowledge regarding these remedies in an easy-to-understand fashion. The book's organization according to ailment makes it very convenient and useful.

Increasing numbers of dissatisfied people are searching for natural remedies that proved their worth long before the advent of "modern medicine."

What is natural healing? It is a way of looking at the world and yourself in relationship with that world. It means that when you experience discomfort or pain, you don't reach for a bottle of pain killers; you search for the cause of that pain, then treat it accordingly, in as noninvasive a manner as possible. Not that drugs do not have their necessary place in medicine's arsenal. The key to natural healing is to become as educated and aware as possible of the many choices available to you.

The days of the omniscient doctor are over. No doctor deserves or should encourage an attitude of blind faith in his patients. Ultimately, one's health is one's own responsibility.

More and more people nowadays are realizing the need to take charge of their own health. Instead of blindly submitting to a physician's orders, they are forming partnerships with their health care providers in which everyone is empowered and responsible. These people are becoming increasingly knowledgeable about their conditions and the various types of treatments available to them.

The Handbook of Natural Folk Remedies offers an excellent array of time-tested folk remedies—foods, herbs, and other nutrients, along with sound and practical advice. It is a valuable aid for anyone who desires to assume more control over his or her own health in a safe, effective way.

Eric S. Roth, MD

Introduction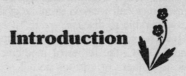

Herbs and other nutritional substances are the oldest form of medicine known to man. While modern, "allopathic" (or conventional) medicine is barely a century old, the practice of natural medicine—using nature as a pharmacy—can be traced back through the civilizations of Rome, Greece, Assyria, Babylon, even to Sumerian times. Over many centuries, man's painstaking experiments with flowers, weeds, plants, roots, leaves, and seeds has yielded a stock of natural medicines to help heal many and varied ailments, almost always without harmful side effects.

We are fortunate to live in an age that offers such high-tech medical solutions as vaccines, antibiotics, laser surgery, and genetic therapy. Today, we would not blow sulfur through a straw into a child's sore throat, swab his neck with kerosene, smear his croupy chest with a messy concoction, blow smoke in his aching ear, or hang little bags of smelly fried onion around his neck to ward off germs (and people who might spread them!).

But we are awakening to the realization that our arsenal of magic bullets comes at a high price. Modern medicine's promise of instant cures—pills or injections that vanquish any bodily ailment—has failed. More and more microbes are becoming resistant to antibiotics, and the AIDS crisis underscores the fact that we have never been able to conquer viruses, even the humble rhinovirus that causes the common cold. Evidence is also mounting in support of the contention made by increasing numbers of physicians and other health care workers that overuse of antibiotics and other symptom-suppressing medicines can weaken immune systems, making us even more vulnerable to disease.

"Let your food be your medicine," said Hippocrates. Between 460 and 370 BC, the father of medicine documented the therapeutic usefulness of various herbal preparations, finally compiling a list of over four hundred herbs and their uses. Dioscorides, physician to Anthony and Cleopatra, left a list of over six hundred healing plants and herbs. By the fifth century, numerous herbals (books on herbal therapy) had been written in various languages. The first truly comprehensive herbal, written in 1597 by English physician John Gerard, was based on research conducted in his own remarkable herb garden. The most extensive studies were conducted by seventeenth-century herbalist Nicholas Culpepper, whose *The Compleat Herbal* is still referenced by modern-day naturopaths and herbalists for its detailed and thorough classification of virtually all known western herbs and their healing properties. Some of those herbs are used in allopathic medicine today.

During the same century in which Culpepper lived and practiced medicine, the first North American settlers carried to the New World the seeds and roots of medicinal, culinary, and fragrant herbs that they had used in Europe. They soon added to their herbal cupboards indigenous plants used by native peoples who were eager to demonstrate their use. Even in frontier days, doctors noted with wonder that Native Americans recovered from wounds that would have proved fatal to the white man. Popular herbs such as anise, slippery elm, sarsaparilla, and red clover—to name only a few—were employed by Native Americans to heal a variety of ailments. Today, we all benefit from Native American medicine, as well as from whatever traditional African medicine survived slavery and colonialism. Those deep traditions of natural healing along with others from literally every corner of the globe have shaped and informed today's lexicon of natural healing remedies.

As more and more ailments defy the best our highly technological allopathic system of medicine has to offer, we are turning increasingly to alternative health caregivers and learning about time-tested natural remedies, revisiting the past in the search for our own solutions.

As we demand greater control over the healing of our own bodies, the allopathic medical community is lagging behind, for the most part choosing to remain uninformed of natural alternatives to prevent and alleviate pain and illness and to effect cures. Patients seeking information are often forced to rely on word-of-mouth, trial-and-error, and whatever tips they glean from books, newspapers, and magazines. This easy-to-use reference book makes that search easier by listing ailments alphabetically, along with their natural remedies, which have been culled from the venerable traditions of many world cultures. It was written to help you achieve the goal of overseeing your own health care, to maintain optimum health in order to prevent disease, as well as to direct you to natural ways in which you can heal common ailments.

Pharmaceutical and natural medicines are not completely distinct. Like pharmaceuticals, herbs are composed of many chemical compounds. In fact, our modern pharmaceutical industry took its original direction from herbal medicine and then emerged as the therapeutic backbone of allopathic medicine. Many commonly used drugs are still derived from the extracts of wild plants, such as aspirin from the willow tree, digitalis from foxglove (which was used by Gypsies for centuries to treat heart troubles), ephedrine from the ma huang bush, morphine and other powerful painkillers from the poppy seed. Many medicines were created after first analyzing herbs, then reproducing the chemistry synthetically. In fact, it is estimated that one out of every four prescription drugs is derived from or patterned after one or more compounds found in medicinal plants. Many researchers admit freely that they use folk medicine and herbology for leads in formulating medicines. However, less than one percent of the 250,000-odd plant species on earth have been studied for medicinal properties. One reason there are so few studies of natural remedies is that such studies cost many millions of dollars. What drug company will underwrite costs for a substance they cannot patent and sell for profit? For example, a small-scale study reported in the *British Medical Journal* showed that when feverfew was dried, powdered, and put in capsules, it effectively reduced the frequency of migraine headaches. It currently costs approximately 231 million dollars to run all the tests and trials required for a new drug to pass the Food and Drug Administration's (FDA) standards for safety and efficacy. If such a study proved that feverfew is an effective migraine treatment, everyone could run out to the health food store to buy it or to a meadow to pick it and prepare a remedy themselves. No one would go to the bother and expense of visiting a medical doctor in order to obtain a prescription for a costly migraine medication.

Another problem is that many drug researchers ignore the fact that herbal properties change according to the season, rainfall, and a host of other variables. In addition, pharmaceutical synthetic reproductions often isolate the active ingredient of the herb, ignoring the possible role of the herb's other properties as either part of the medicinal effect or a counter to possible side effects.

On the other hand, too many people assume that herbs either have a beneficial effect or no effect at all. The truth is that many herbs exert powerful effects, and though they generally do not create the kind of negative side effects associated with allopathic medicines, if they are not used properly, they can be dangerous.

Overall, the history of human use of herbal medicine is long and effective, but, in recent times, sadly underexplored, particularly in the United States. In Asia and Europe, on the other hand, researchers and manufacturers are redefining health food, packing food products with disease-fighting nutrients and herbs. Relax Time chewing gum, for example, releases extracts of the herb valerian, which promotes sleep and acts as a natural tranquilizer. Some snack foods are supplemented with echinacea, an herb that stimulates the immune system and helps it fight disease. Under the FDA's strict regulations, these revolutionary health foods are considered pharmaceuticals that must undergo extensive and expensive trials before being approved. They will probably never be sold in the US.

Yet, the tide may be turning in favor of less expensive, natural alternative medicines. As health-care costs continue to escalate, more attention is finally being paid to preventive medicine, to preserving the natural plants that give us medicines, and to natural ways of strengthening and healing our bodies. Big-name pharmaceutical companies are now branching out into botanicals. New companies specializing in plant-derived drugs are springing up. Recently, Pfizer, Inc., teamed up with the New York Botanical Garden to collect and study plants for healing properties. The Merck Company, which also collaborates with the New York Botanical Garden, recently found a chemical in a plant from the ginger family that holds promise as an antiparasitic drug. And a possible cancer treatment derived from the camptotheca plant may evolve from SmithKline Beecham's teamwork with the Morrow Arboretum at the University of Pennsylvania in Philadelphia. Only a few years ago, the federal government gave a tacit stamp of approval to herbal medicines when the FDA authorized the sale of herbal teas made by Traditional Medicinals of Rohnert Park, California, as remedies for colds, insomnia, obesity, and other problems. That decision and others like it confirm what devotees of herbal cures have long believed—that nature's time-honored medicines can cure or help to cure many maladies, as well as bolster immunity. We are beginning to rediscover that a humble vegetable, fruit, weed, leaf, flower, bark, root, or seed can offer a solution, after all.

It is important to keep in mind that not all natural healers or herbalists are equally effective. Some of those who dub themselves natural healers are unaware of the full properties of the remedies they prescribe and under what conditions these substances should be used. Many patented herbal remedies and healers also focus unduly on the detoxifying properties of herbal medicine. Weaker patients can become ill from overly heavy detoxification. These "healers" fail to recognize that certain herbs build and tonify the body, as well as balance overall circulation, increasing activity in some areas and decreasing it in others. A balance must be struck between building and cleansing the body, and it takes skill and experience to gauge how far to tip the balance either way for an individual patient. A good herbalist will help the patient eliminate toxins and build strength as needed. Herbalists should also counsel patients that while healing through natural means is a lengthier process, it is also less apt to bring with it harmful side effects.

None of the recipes given in the following pages will cause harm if taken in reasonable quantities. It is always advisable, however, to obtain a professional diagnosis as to the cause of any ailment that persists for more than a week or two. For the treatment of serious ailments, seek out a trained herbalist for consultation concerning the remedies included in this book.

But you don't have to wait for illness to strike to use many of the herbs recommended here. Begin introducing them into your regular diet as a preventative measure. One way is to add herbs to lemonade or to brew teas. In Europe, people brew herb teas to drink every day as preventative or healing measures. Some popular herbs for everyday use are chamomile (for stress, nerves, indigestion), peppermint (a good digestive, counter to chills, and overall stimulant), thyme (same as peppermint plus eases mountain sickness), coneflower (boosts immune system), evening primrose (eases insomnia, PMS), licorice (helpful against ulcers, liver conditions, and a great blood cleanser and complexion clearer), lime flowers (for insomnia), elderflower (for chills), rosemary (for headaches), and milk thistle (protection against liver ailments like cirrhosis and hepatitis). Culinary herbs such as oregano, sage, and rosemary can be used in cooking. Europeans also concoct syrups, such as elderberry rob, the juice of the fruit heated and sweetened, and thyme-linseed syrup to treat coughs and colds.

You will find that many of the ingredients used to make these folk remedies are already in your refrigerator or cupboard. Other ingredients will require a trip to your local health food store. Another useful source is the many mail order companies specializing in health products that are listed in the back of magazines on natural healing.

In many instances, the list of treatments for a particular ailment is lengthy and varied. Choose the remedies that appeal to you or contain ingredients that are most convenient to obtain and use.

Part of the fun of becoming your own herbalist is experimenting to discover which cures are best for you, your family, and friends. Self-treating minor injuries and common illnesses will give you a wonderful sense of empowerment and control over your body. It also connects you with a venerable tradition practiced for thousands of years, all over the world. And the beauty of these cures and remedies is they are cost-effective and can be used in the privacy of your own home.

"Nature is the healer of all disease," Hippocrates stated thousands of years ago. Aristotle, another wise Greek, advised, "If there is one way better than another, it is the way of nature."

Herbs Commonly Used

The following is a list of popular herbs, spices, and other nutritional ingredients found in many natural remedies. They were used either by Native Americans or brought here by the peoples of Africa, Asia, and Europe. Unless you have a chronic or recurring condition that requires you to always have a particular herb on hand, it is best to purchase—or pick—these herbs as needed, in order to ensure maximum freshness and potency.

Alfalfa (*Medicago sativa*)—an extremely rich herb when it comes to nutrients, alfalfa is particularly high in betacarotene, vitamins B2, B6, C, D, and K. It is also an important source of chlorophyll. It helps to lower cholesterol by binding to it and preventing it from being absorbed by the body. Since alfalfa contains eight different digestive enzymes, it helps regulate the PH of the stomach, thus balancing stomach contents and improving digestion in people prone to acidity. Make this herb part of your daily diet by using fresh alfalfa sprouts as a garnish and in mixed salads.

Anise (*Pimpinella anisum*)—this is among the most ancient herbs; it appeared in an Egyptian herbal written in 1500 BC. Brought to America by the first settlers, it has been popular in American herb gardens ever since. Chewed after meals, anise seeds improve digestion and eliminate flatulence. Available in the whole or ground seed, tincture, and tea, anise is also effective in cough remedies because of its pleasant flavor and expectorant properties.

Arnica (*Arnica montana*)—tincture of arnica (also known as mountain tobacco) is used in a liquid or ointment that is applied to sprains and bruises. It must not be taken internally, except in homeopathic form.

Astralagus (*Astralagus membranaceus*)—used by Oriental herbalists, astralagus stimulates immune action and combats heart disease. Studies show that it boosts the numbers and activity of white blood cells that eliminate bacteria and viruses. It also destroys mutant cells that may become cancerous. The herb's main contribution may lie in its ability to stimulate the production of interferon and thereby increase the immune system's effectiveness in fighting disease. One study reported that the herb decreased incidence of colds and cut the length of viral illnesses in half. Astralagus is available in patented Chinese formula medicines and by itself in capsules and tinctures.

Bilberry (*Vaccinium myrtillus*)—a natural antioxidant, in Europe it is used to treat varicose veins and for problems with blood circulation to the brain. Bilberry also inhibits blood platelet aggregation (clotting). It helps to improve a wide range of eye problems such as night blindness, photophobia, glaucoma, and diabetic retinopathy. When combined with vitamin E, it stopped the progression of cataracts in 97 percent of fifty patients suffering from cortical cataracts. Bilberry is available in capsules and tinctures.

Boneset (or Feverwort) (*Eupatorium perfoliatum*)—the leaves and flowers of this weed can be brewed as a tea or a decoction to make an extremely helpful fever reducer. It is also available in capsules and tinctures.

Borage (*Borago officinalis*)—the leaves of this plant with exquisite blue starlike flowers taste like cucumber and have been used since the early days of the Greeks for a wide variety of ailments, particularly for depression and nervous tension. It is a rich source of calcium and potassium, two minerals important to the nervous system and for calming and strengthening the heart. It also tones and stimulates the adrenal glands. In France, a tea is made by pouring boiling water on one ounce of fresh or dried leaves and used for alleviation of fevers and pulmonary complaints. Borage oil, taken in capsule form or as part of a compound supplement, is widely recognized today for its effectiveness against the symptoms of menopause.

Burdock Root (*Arctium lappa*)—this nutritional herb is used in herbal blood-purifying mixtures. The Japanese and people who follow a macrobiotic diet boil the roots in salted water and eat them with sauce. Country Russian folk claim that a broth prepared from burdock root prevents hair loss and stimulates its growth. Burdock helps the body eliminate excess uric acid, which may benefit some types of arthritis and gout. It's rich in nutrients and helps the body replace minerals lost in diuresis. Burdock also helps relieve lymphatic congestion and improve many types of skin conditions. During the Industrial Revolution, burdock root was consumed as a vegetable and a tea to help people better cope with air pollutants. German research shows that burdock contains polyacetylenes that kill bacteria and fungi. Burdock root is available in tea, capsule and tincture forms. It can also be purchased fresh at some Oriental and health food stores and prepared like any other root vegetable.

Calendula (or Marigold) (*Calendula officinalis*)—stimulating to the digestion, calendula is high in vitamins A and C. A hot tea made from these flowers is excellent for circulation and a good tuner for the immune system. Topically, an ointment or balm made from calendula makes a wonderful remedy for skin disorders and an excellent antiseptic for cuts and inflammations of any kind.

Cardamom (*Elettaria cardomomum*)—this East Indian spice is a staple in curry powder, but the seeds are an effective after-meal breath sweetener and stimulant to the digestion. The oil is especially invigorating when added to bath water.

Cat's claw (*Uncaria tomentosa*)—this woody vine from the rain forests of Peru is being hailed currently as a wonder remedy for an amazing range and variety of illnesses and is distributed in the United States in capsule, tea, tincture, and tablet forms. The medicinal properties are found in the inner bark of the vine and in the root, but the Peruvian government forbids harvest of the root in order to ensure survival of this valuable plant species. The herb is a powerful cellular reconstitutor, with applications in the treatment of cancer, arthritis, gastritis, ulcers, rheumatism, irregularities of the female cycle, acne, organic depression, allergies, neurobronchitis, genital herpes, herpes zoster, a wide variety of infections, tumors, cysts, chronic fatigue syndrome, shingles dysbiosis, Crohn's disease, and the opportunistic infections that plague AIDS patients. Topically, it is excellent for the treatment of wounds, fungus, fistulas, hemorrhoids, and other health problems. Interest in cat's claw began in the early 70's, when it was reported that a Peruvian plantation owner had been cured of terminal cancer after drinking cat's claw tea daily over a six-month period. Since he was of Austrian descent, word spread quickly to Europe, where studies continue to show this herb's amazing versatility in treating an apparently endless list of bodily ailments. The consensus seems to be that 3 to 6 grams daily in divided doses is therapeutic if using tablets or capsules, three to four cups of tea, or twenty to thirty drops, three or four times a day, if using liquid extract. Based on research, cat's claw seems to be a powerful adaptogen suitable for long-term use in both chronic and acute conditions. However, studies of this recently discovered (at least to North American and European herbalists) remedy have not been conducted long enough to completely dispel the possibility of side effects. It is available loose and dried, in capsules, pills, and tinctures.

Catnip—this versatile, age-old herb calms upset tummies, relieves nervous headaches, and promotes fever-cooling perspiration. It has even been used to silence hiccups and persistent coughs. The Pennsylvania Dutch give the delicious mint tea made from catnip to babies and small children to aid digestion and promote a restful sleep. Catnip is most effective in combination with chamomile and peppermint. However, be aware that in excessive doses it can produce nausea. It is available as a tea and in capsules and tinctures.

Cayenne Pepper—cayenne contains a high vitamin C content. This versatile condiment provides effective treatment for many maladies. But it is best known for its ability to stimulate metabolism and lower triglycerides. Cayenne is being studied currently for its possible healing effect on several ailments, including ulcers and stomach cancers. Cayenne also makes a great spice for almost any meal. It is available ground and in capsules.

Celery (*Apium graveolens*)—in ancient times, celery was considered a medicine rather than a food. Hippocrates prescribed it as a diuretic, and it still is used for that purpose today. It is a valuable remedy for arthritis, rheumatism, lumbago, and nervous tension.

Chamomile (*Chamaemelum nobile*)—chamomile is actually the best medicine for a garden. Nothing benefits ailing plants as much as sprinkling this herb ''doctor'' over their beds. Chamomile contains calcium in an easily absorbed form, plus a volatile oil and glucoside with relaxing qualities. All of this makes chamomile a wonderful natural tranquilizer that soothes both the nerves and the digestive tract. It also boasts natural antibiotic properties. The Romans used it for a bitter tonic and blood purifier, the French drink it after meals to aid digestion and boil it to make a compress for piles. Women drink it for menstrual cramps and to bring on delayed menstruation. Chamomile tea, made by pouring one pint of boiling water over an ounce of the flowers, is an old remedy for hysteria. Chamomile steam baths are said to ease difficulty in elderly men's urination. Chamomile is also used to relieve flatulence, as a tonic, and to relieve neck and ear pains due to swollen glands. It is also used as a children's remedy to relieve and prevent nightmares and gas pains. Bags of chamomile flowers, steeped in boiling water, can be used as poultices for various skin problems, including facial swellings caused by abscesses. If you're allergic to ragweed pollen, avoid chamomile, as they are from the same botanical family. Chamomile is available loose and dried, in tea bags, capsules, tinctures, and some cosmetics and creams.

Chapparal (*Laurea divaricatum*)—this American-Indian herb cleanses the blood, boosts the immune system, combats urinary tract infections and kidney stones, relieves skin rashes, and helps fight cancer. It is available as a tea, in capsules and tinctures.

Comfrey (*Aymphytum officinale*)—three thousand years ago, the Greeks used this valuable herb for a wide variety of ailments. Research indicates that comfrey's active ingredient is allantoin, a substance that is soluble in hot water. Allantoin is also found in the urine of pregnant women and plants, indicating that its function is related to growth. Modern herbalists caution against comfrey's internal use, as it is said to speed cell growth and therefore might have carcinogenic properties. But applied as a poultice, comfrey is known to promote the knitting of bone and aid the healing of joint and cartilage injuries, as well as swellings and bruises when applied as fomentations. Comfrey poultices help to heal severe cuts, boils, abscesses, and gangrenous ulcers. Comfrey is available loose and dried and in tinctures.

Corn silk (*Zea mays* or *Stigmata maidis*)—the yellowish, fine "threads" that cover the "ear" of the corn were a popular remedy for bladder complaints in the old days and later were prescribed by doctors as a diuretic and to relieve cystitis and even gonorrhea. Corn silk is available as a tea, in capsules and tinctures.

Damiana (*Turnera diffusa*)—this plant grows wild in Southern California, Mexico, and Texas, and its chemical composition is not entirely known. The Indians indigenous to the above areas have used damiana leaves since antiquity to relieve nervous and muscular weakness. In turn-of-the-century America, the fluid extract of damiana or pills made from the leaves were even used as a remedy for impotence. Scientists generally agree that damiana has a general tonic effect on the reproductive organs, and, as such, is a *bona fide* aphrodisiac and a nervous system strengthener. Damiana is available in capsules and tinctures.

Dandelion (*Taraxacum officinale*)—though dandelion originated in Greece, it has spread throughout the world. The root of this valuable roadside plant can be taken as a tea or the leaves eaten in salads. It can also be steamed or lightly sauteed. As is the case with all vegetables, overcooking or boiling in large amounts of water for long periods will strip it of valuable nutrients. Rich in vitamins A (richest in A than any leafy green except violet leaves), B1, and C, dandelion contains more iron than spinach, and is full of purifying agents. The leaves and roots make an excellent tonic for the kidneys, liver, spleen, pancreas, and urinary tract. The entire plant contains nutritive salts that act as a blood cleanser, often with amazing speed. In old-time rural America, dandelion roots were roasted slowly, then pulverized, and used as a coffee substitute that is said to prevent the formation of gallstones. Dandelion "coffee," a healthful beverage with no caffeine, is sold today in health food stores.

Dong quai—this Asian root is used often as a blood purifier, circulation booster, skin softener, and as a tonic treatment for female complaints such as menopause, as well as menstrual discomfort. Dong quai is available in Chinese patent medicine formulas, as well as by itself in capsules and tinctures.

Echinacea (*Echinacea species*)—extracted from the purple coneflower, a daisylike plant common to the American plains, Echinacea heightens immunity by stimulating stem cells in bone marrow and lymphatic tissue. It cleanses the lymph system and stimulates and supports the immune system, helping to eliminate bacteria, germs, and cancer-causing substances from the blood.

Elderflower and Berries (*Sambucus canadensis or S. nigra*)—this herb grows wild in North America and is used all over the world. Elder is said to be most effective when the flowers and berries are picked at high noon. Elderflowers have traditionally been administered as a tea for treatment of lung infections, measles, and scarlet fever. Elder blossom tea is an effective fever reducer that promotes perspiration. It also has a mild stimulating effect. Elderflower water is a commonly used astringent and skin smoother. The delicately flavored blossoms can also be added to cakes, muffins, or pancakes. The berries are somewhat laxative and have been used throughout the ages for rheumatism and arthritis. The flowers and the berries are available in loose and dried form, in capsules, in tinctures, and the berries are also made into a healthful, delicious wine or a syrup considered helpful for sore throats and asthma.

Eucalyptus—this herb is mainly grown in Australia, but we in North America use it so much that we import it by the ton. Almost all commercial throat and cough remedies, as well as nasal sprays, contain eucalyptus. Its effect is to cool but it is actually working as a mild irritant that produces heat and promotes circulation.

Evening primrose oil (*Primula vulgaris*)—until recently viewed as a wild weed, the oil from evening primrose seeds is highly effective against inflammation and swelling, and it can soothe arthritic joints. Recent research indicates that this oil, taken in capsule form, is extremely effective for a number of health problems, particularly PMS and other inflammatory conditions associated with female problems.

Fennel (*Foeniculum vulgare*)—for many centuries this seed, grown mainly in Asia minor, has been esteemed both as a culinary and medicinal herb, especially in treating eye ailments. The Greeks gave fennel to their athletes as a food when competing in the Olympic games, because it strengthened them without making them fat. Fennel tea is made with bruised fennel seeds. Most recipes call for the simultaneous use of fennel with catnip, especially for indigestion. In more superstitious times, it was customary to hang up bunches of fennel in the home as a protection against evil spirits, and those in fear of ghosts stuffed the keyholes of their doors with fennel seeds.

Fenugreek (*Foenum graecum*)—this tasty herb was first prized by the ancient peoples of Asia and those who lived on the shores of the Mediterranean as a valuable antipollutant for the body. However, fenugreek seeds make a tea that is a wonderful natural medicine for an impressive array of ailments, including blood poisoning, bowel irritation, constipation, low libido, flatulence, and high cholesterol. It is perhaps most prized for helping the body rid itself of excess mucus and trapped toxins.

Feverfew (*Tanacetum parthenium*)—nature's headache and fever remedy is a bushy perennial that belongs to the daisy family of plants and is a close cousin to echinacea, burdock, and calendula. Feverfew is a remarkable example of medical science learning from folk medicine. In 1633, the famous English herbalist Gerard wrote of feverfew's effectiveness for "them that are giddy in the head, and for the 'St. Anthony's fire,' to all inflammations and hot swellings." In 1772, John Hill, MD, wrote in his *Family Herbal*, "in the worst headache, this herb exceeds whatever else is known."

Feverfew is fast becoming one of the most sought-after alternative medicines for pain relief, with an effect similar to that of aspirin. The active constituents identified in feverfew inhibit the production of prostaglandins, chemical substances present in the body in minute amounts that are involved in the inflammatory process. But feverfew has demonstrated its effectiveness, without aspirin's side effects. This herb also possesses ingredients that inhibit leukotriences, slow-reacting substances that stimulate allergic reactions. Among feverfew's other benefits are relief from sinus and allergy discomfort, psoriasis, spondylosis, menstrual cramps, menopause, allergies, high blood pressure, and spinal problems. It is available in loose, dried form, tea bags, capsules, and tinctures.

Figs (*Ficus carica*)—the laxative properties of this fruit have been prized since the days of the early Egyptians and Greeks, who first cultivated the trees. Figs are also valued for their ability to restore the vitality of those who are ill for a lengthy period and, generally, for their high nutritional content. The Spanish brought fig trees to North America, and by the end of the sixteenth century, many varieties were thriving here.

Flaxseed (Lindseed) (*Linum usitatissimum*)—one of the oldest crops, flax dates back as early as 5000 BC. Flax seeds, together with cloth woven from linen thread, have been found in Egyptian tombs. Flax flowers are usually blue and contain the mucilaginous seed called flaxseed. Flaxseed is often added to cough mixtures, and the tea with honey and lemon juice is a good folk remedy for coughs and colds. The oil derived from this seed is a rich source of the essential fatty acids (EFAs), especially omega 3/linoleic acid, which help form the cell membrane that surrounds every cell in the human body. EFAs are also required for the transport and metabolism of both cholesterol and triglycerides. They can lower high cholesterol levels up to 25 percent and high triglyceride levels up to 65 percent. EFAs also help form hormonelike substances called prostaglandins, which are necessary for the regulation of virtually every function in the human body. These functions include regulating platelet stickiness, arterial muscle tone, inflammatory response, sodium excretion through the kidney, and immune function. The Cherokee Indians mixed flaxseed oil with either goat or moose milk, honey, and pumpkin to nourish pregnant and nursing mothers. It was also given to people with skin diseases, arthritis, malnutrition, and as a tonic for virility. They believed that flax oil captured energies from the sun that could then be released and used in the body's metabolism.

Flaxseed oil can be added to salads, vegetables, soups, and rice. Daily recommendation is one to two tablespoons at the same meal with protein. It can also be taken in capsule form.

Garlic (*Allium sativum*)—this pungent bulb, a close relative of the onion, has a history of service to mankind as ancient and honorable as that of any plant. The intense smell of garlic is so penetrating that it is exhaled in the breath of anyone who has even had a clove of it applied to the soles of his feet.

Garlic is among the best-researched of all herbs. Its active properties lie in an essential oil, sulphide of allyl, which is rich in sulphur and present in all members of the onion family. Renowned for its ability to lower high blood pressure, garlic is also effective as a blood thinner, aid to circulation, detoxifier, and natural antibiotic and antihistamine. It also lowers cholesterol and triglycerides in the blood, preventing blood clots by blocking the formation of thromboxane, a clotting factor, and lowering the levels of fibrinogen, another contributor to clotting. Studies have shown that garlic contains eighteen antiviral, antifungal, and bacterial substances. It also seems to be a powerful cancer fighter, particularly against stomach and colon cancers. F. Gilbert McMahon, MD, and a group of researchers at Tulane University in Louisiana, discovered that total cholesterol and low-density (bad) cholesterol are reduced after a twelve week regime of one and a half cloves of garlic or a 900-milligram capsule of powdered garlic daily. Elise Malecki, PhD, a researcher at Penn State, reports a strong link between garlic and lowered risk of colon cancer. She also points to the low incidence of stomach cancer in areas in China where garlic is consumed heavily. New York Hospital–Cornell Medical Center in New York City established a Garlic Information Center to help spread the word about the role of garlic and garlic supplements in preventing and treating infections, heart disease, and certain types of cancer.

Gentian root (*Gentiana lutea*)—not all the many varieties of this root are medicinal. One that is most used in healing remedies is the yellow-flowered gentian. In ancient times, this root was used for weakness, fatigue, stomach troubles, liver problems, and as an antidote to some poisons.

Ginger (*Zingiber officinale*)—the root of the ginger is a stimulant, tending to excite the glands to action. Though most renowned for its ability to relieve nausea and digestive distress, ginger's ability to bring heat and circulation to any area of the body makes it a favorite of people around the world for combating colds and flu, drawing out toxins and gas, loosening mucus in the throat and bronchial tubes, promoting menstruation, and restoring appetites. Much like aspirin, but without the side effects, ginger inhibits thromboxanes and platelet aggregation, helping to prevent strokes and heart failure. If the whole root is not available, you can find ginger in capsules and tinctures.

Gingko biloba (*Ginkgo biloba*)—the ginkgo biloba tree is the oldest surviving species of tree on earth. Ginkgo trees survived the Ice Age, but only on the Asian continent, where it has a centuries-old history of effectiveness against many ailments, particularly such age-related complaints as poor circulation, short-term memory loss, fatigue, and general mental deterioration. Gingko wasn't known to Europe until the seventeenth century, but is being actively researched today for its ability to aid the brain's ability to utilize oxygen and glucose more efficiently, increase general circulation by increasing blood vessel flexibility, and improve the rate at which information is transmitted at the nerve level.

This herb is most effective when you use extract of gingko leaf, as it is currently widely prescribed in Europe, and increasingly, here in North America. Gingko also inhibits the production of PAF (platelet activation factor), a substance produced by the body and involved in a tremendous number of biological processes such as organ graft rejection, asthma attacks, blood clots involved in heart attacks, and some strokes. Recent studies show that ginkgo also helps to relieve impotence caused by arterial erectile dysfunction, as well as those with high HDL (high-density lipoprotein) cholesterol. Gingko is usually taken in capsules and extracts.

Ginseng (*Panax ginseng*)—this is another well-known herb, with many claims made for its healing abilities. Research suggests it promotes homeostasis, maintaining steady blood pressure, blood sugar, and energy levels. Ginseng is found in North America but it was popularized by Asians who have used the root for over five thousand years to boost energy levels, counteract aging, tone the respiratory tract, and improve sexual function. Overall, ginseng strengthens the entire endocrine system and sets the metabolism at a more efficient level. Do not take it at night because of its stimulating properties. Use the expensive roots, as they are less apt to irritate.

Siberian ginseng (Eleutherococcus senticosus) is a close relative of panax ginseng, but is actually not a true ginseng. It does energize the entire bodily system, and it relieves stress and fatigue without side effects. Siberian ginseng also increases endurance and works as an adaptogen to help the body acclimate to mental and physical stress. Because it is said to contain testosterone, it is useful in treating impotence. Ginseng root can be purchased in Oriental pharmacies and some health food and herbal stores. It is more commonly available in capsule, pill, tea, and tincture forms.

Goldenseal root (*Laurea divaricatum*)—a powerful natural antibiotic used externally and internally to fight all types of infection, goldenseal is used alone and in combination with other herbs. It should not be used by those suffering from high blood pressure or by anyone for longer than seven days in succession. Goldenseal is available in powder form, in capsules and tinctures. Because of its intensely bitter taste, most people prefer to use the capsules.

Green tea—recent research has found that drinking green tea (or taking capsules) helps prevent heart disease, reduces the risk of cancer, fights the flu, lowers blood sugar, and limits the growth of bacteria that cause cavities and dental plaque. These varied health benefits come from its rich supply of plant chemicals called polyphenols.

Hawthorn berry, leaves, and flowers (*Crataegus oxyacantha*)—this safe herb is used in Europe to lower cholesterol and tone heart action. Hawthorn berries are naturally high in flavenoids and help to dilate blood vessels, thereby increasing coronary blood flow, protecting against oxygen deficiency, and preventing irregular heartbeat, which can cause heart attacks. Studies also indicate that it acts as a calcium channel blocker. Hawthorn also helps to decrease fatty acids and lactic acids in the body. It is available in loose and dried form, in capsules and tinctures.

Honey—a natural antibiotic and soft tissue emulcent with soothing and healing properties, honey is an essential ingredient in countless remedies for both external and internal ailments.

Hops (*Humulus lupulus*)—this native North American plant is cultivated for its cones, which are used medicinally and in making beer and ale (which, for some conditions, can also be viewed as medicinal). Centuries ago, hop pickers were the first to notice that the strong aroma of the plant soothes nerves. It also relieves indigestion and insomnia.

Horehound (*Marrubium vulgare*)—a venerable herb once thought to cure a myriad of ills, horehound leaf is commonly used today for its soothing and expectorant properties in cough drops and syrup formulas.

Horseradish Root—like the humble onion, garlic, and cayenne, horseradish is considered a food rather than a medicinal herb. But like its nutritional compatriots, its considerable healing powers have made it a popular natural medicine for many cultures throughout history. Horseradish is effective for a variety of problems, both internal and external, including colds, flus, and coughs, neuralgia, and bloating due to malfunctioning kidneys. It is taken raw, usually grated and mixed with food or drunk as a tea.

Hyssop (*Hyssopus officinalis*)—this versatile herb is particularly valuable taken as a tea in cases of chronic catarrh, chest troubles, and rheumatism. It is also available in capsules and tinctures.

Juniper (*Juniperus communis*)—the tree bears fruit which appear to resemble berries rather than cones, and it is these juniper ''berries'' which yield the volatile oil used in medicine and the production of gin. Distilled oil of juniper or decoctions made from the berries are used as diuretics and carminatives in the treatment of diseases of the kidney and bladder and to alleviate indigestion. In France, it is also prescribed for chest complaints. It is available in loose and dried form, in capsules and tinctures.

Jujube dates (*genus Zizyphus*)—these dates are a sedative and a tonic. They help relax the smooth muscles and are considered a tonic for the nervous system. In Oriental medicine, jujube dates are used for weakness, shortness of breath and irritability.

Lady's slipper (*Cypripedium pubescens*)—this wild orchid is found everywhere from North America through Latin America and India. The root of this flower is one of the safest and most beneficial plants for the nervous system, and it is commonly used in combination with other herbs such as balm and scullcap in teas, capsules, and tincture formulas.

Licorice root (*Glycrrhiza glabra*)—known as "the great harmonizer" in Chinese medicine, licorice root is often added to herbal formulas, in part for its sweetening properties. It is an excellent anti-inflammatory agent, helps to speed the healing of ulcers, and is supportive to the adrenal glands. It is included in many cough formulas to soothe irritated mucous membranes and is often found in cough lozenges and pastilles. The sugar of licorice is said to be safe for diabetic sufferers. In some countries, it is even employed to promote female fertility. A drink made from one ounce of the peeled and bruised root, infused in one pint of boiling water for five or ten minutes, is useful in cases of sore throat and of catarrhal conditions occuring in the urinary and intestinal tracts. Many people chew on the root, both to stimulate the gums and to combat oral cravings associated with quitting the cigarette habit. Licorice can also increase energy levels and muscle tone. **Note**: Do not use if you have high blood pressure.

Marshmallow (*Althea officinalis*)—Charlemagne cultivated the leaves and roots of this perennial herb within his empire because of its ability to heal irritated mucus membranes in the digestive, urinary, and respiratory tracts. It is generally prescribed along with other herbs for bronchitis and coughs, and the powdered roots are also commonly used as a healing poultice on inflamed areas.

Boiled in wine or milk, marshmallow was once a popular remedy for coughs, bronchitis, and similar respiratory troubles. It is available loose and dried, in capsules and tinctures.

Milk thistle (*Silybum marianum*)—an extract of the common milk thistle weed strengthens and stimulates the liver, helping it to synthesize quality fats such as phospholipids and to improve protein synthesis and the quality of blood protein. Milk thistle can even rebuild livers damaged by alcohol, drugs, hepatitis or cirrhosis. Strengthening the liver is essential for overall health, disease resistance, and for cancer prevention. The active ingredient in milk thistle is a flavenoid called silymarin. The seeds also contain large amounts of linoleic acid. Milk thistle works best over an extended period of time.

Motherwort (*Leonurus cardiaca*)—this perennial plant was imported from Europe and Asia to North America specifically because of its healing qualities. Traditionally known as the "herb of life," the Japanese dedicate one of their four major annual festivals to motherwort. Long esteemed as a heart tonic, modern scientists have discovered that the herb is rich in calcium chloride, which is necessary for a healthy heart. It is also considered beneficial to the entire nervous system, a tonic and cooler to the female organs, and it is useful in treating difficult menopause.

Mushrooms—long a crucial part of Oriental medicine, many health researchers consider various fungi to be among the most healthful foods available. Studies show that ganoderma lucidum, known as *reishi* in Japan and *ling zhe* in China, has antitumor properties and stimulates the immune system. It is also a voracious free radical scavenger, normalizes blood pressure, and lowers cholesterol. In the Orient, reishi is regarded as a symbol of youth and longevity and is even called "the plant of immortality." Those with rheumatoid arthritis and varicose veins have all reported help from this mushroom.

Shiitake and enoki mushroons are popular heart-protective and anticancer fungi.

Nettles (*Urtica dioica*)—as a folk remedy for the relief of asthma, the leaves were dried and burned and the smoke inhaled. The Romans prepared a healing ointment by steeping the leaves in vegetable oil. In Russia, the plant is used to relieve toothache and sciatica, while in Jamaica, nettle juice is dropped into open wounds. The North Indians used it for urinary problems and to stop bleeding. In Germany and Russia, rural folk rub or strike rheumatic body parts with bundles of fresh nettles for several minutes. With its high vitamin C content, this highly nutritious herb is beneficial in alleviating congestion, allergies, and hay fever. It is particularly strengthening to the kidneys and its high iron content makes it an excellent blood-builder. Nettle soup and nettle tea make excellent alkaline spring tonics to perk up livers made sluggish by rich wintertime foods. Nettle is also a well-known diuretic and can relieve rheumatism and gout in the elderly. It is available as a tea, in capsules, and tinctures.

Oats (*Avena sativa*)—wild oat extract is rich in many nutrients and has been used to increase muscle mass and stamina. Oats also contain tissue-soothing ingredients that make it excellent against both internal and external irritation.

Onion—the onion is one of the oldest vegetables known to man. In early times, people would place slices of onion around the home, believing that its pungent aroma would ward off evil spirits and diseases. In fact, some people follow this custom today, destroying the peeled, bruised, or cut bulb (and whatever diseases it has trapped) after a few hours. That practice may have sound science behind it. Researchers have discovered that onions produce an electrical field similar to that produced by penicillin. However, most herbalists prefer to use the onion. The juice is an effective diuretic, and when diluted with honey, it helps to bring up coughs and heal colds. This versatile bulb is said to lower blood pressure and help restore sexual potency. Studies have shown that the onion, like garlic, decreases blood cholesterol levels—even after eating a fatty meal—and it can also fight off excessive platelet aggregation, which can lead to clotting in the bloodstream. You will discover in this book that this simple vegetable is useful for an amazing variety of ailments. However, do not overeat onions. In an experiment, soldiers ate two pounds of onions every day. After five days, all showed symptoms of anemia.

Parsley (*Petroselinum crispum*)—this herb was used in ancient times for many illnesses, particularly those affecting the bladder and kidneys, and to dissolve kidney stones. Early herbalists wrote that the use of parsley would "fasten loose teeth, brighten dim eyes, and relieve a stitch in the side." We know today that parsley is extremely rich in vitamins A and C. Parsley tea was utilized in World War I, when men in the trenches developed kidney trouble and dysentery. In France, an ointment made from green parsley and snails was a popular application for scrofulous swellings, and the bruised leaves have been applied externally to tumors. Yet parsley is used today mainly as a garnish that is left behind after the dish it decorated is consumed and to overcome the strong odor of garlic.

Make parsley a staple of your daily diet. You can add chopped parsley to soups, broths, egg and vegetable dishes, salad dressings, and eat it with hamburger, meat loaf, fish, and many other dishes. One-half cup of chopped parsley added to a four-pound stew provides up to ten thousand units of vitamin A alone. It is also available in capsule form.

Peppermint (*Mentna piperita*—the oil of this herb relieves stress, anxiety, and frayed nerves. Its main ingredient, menthol, is recognized by the FDA as a medicine. A proven painkiller and counterirritant, peppermint also relieves gas, nausea, and other digestive upsets. The tea is wonderful for upset tummies, especially mixed with chamomile. Peppermint is similar to spearmint, but much stronger, so children with upset stomachs should be given spearmint tea instead.

Plantain (*Plantago major*)—this flowering plant has been used as a healing agent since the days of the ancient Greeks for wounds, external ulcers, coughs, and colds. The Anglo-Saxons bound the crushed leaves to their heads to relieve headaches. It was used by the North American Indians for a wide variety of ailments, among them insect stings, sores, rheumatism, burns, swellings, rattlesnake bites, and colds, coughs, and fevers. It is available in loose and dried form, in teas, capsules, and tinctures.

Raspberry leaf (*Rubus spp.*)—high in vitamin C and many minerals, this tea is an excellent remedy for colds if taken when symptoms first show themselves. It is also wonderfully supportive for pregnant women. Raspberry is also available in capsules.

Red clover (*Trifolium pratense*)—a remedy for colds and coughs, red clover acts as a mild sedative to encourage sleep, purify the blood, and enhance the immune system. Red clover tea is also effective for all kinds of intestinal distress, and its demulcent qualities soothe the pain of intestinal ulcers. The blossoms contain calcium and phosphorous, necessary for strong bones and teeth. It is also available in loose and dried form, capsules and tinctures.

Rosemary (*Rosmarinus officinalis*)—the ancients claimed that this mint strengthened the memory. Today it is still considered a mild brain stimulant that sharpens memory, alertness, and concentration. In the Middle Ages, the young tops, leaves, and flowers were infused into a tea that was used for nervousness, convulsions, liver troubles, headache, and stomach disorders. Mixed with honey to make a syrup, it relieved bronchitis and asthma. A liniment prepared from the herb was used for rheumatism and pain. It is also commonly prescribed by herbalists as an effective heart tonic and as a remedy against high blood pressure, headaches, and the threat of miscarriage. It is also used for conditions of the skin and scalp. Rosemary wine is made by chopping up sprigs of green rosemary and soaking them in white wine, which is strained off after a few days. It stimulates the brain and nervous system. Rosemary tea, made by infusing one ounce of flowering tops in a pint of boiling water, is good for headaches, colds, colics, and nervous troubles. It is also available in loose and dried form, capsules, tinctures, and oil.

Sage (*Salvia officinalis*)—we know sage today mostly as a culinary herb used in poultry dressings and sauces for fish. But in the Middle Ages, sage was used for almost every ailment, particularly those associated with the spleen. The centuries-old practice of using sage when cooking rich meats such as pork and goose has good sense behind it, because the herb is a digestive. This common plant is still highly regarded as a medicinal herb today. The health-giving and palatable tea (made by the infusion of a handful of fresh leaves in a pint of boiling water) is an effective gargle for bleeding gums, sore throats, and tonsilitis. The plant makes a good healing poultice for ulcers, sores, and skin eruptions, and its astringent properties help stop bleeding. Red sage, though harder to come by, is considered the more effective variety. Sage is available in loose and dried form, capsules, and tinctures.

Sarsaparilla (*Smilax officinalis*)—the dried root of this evergreen shrub was a popular medicine among the American Indians and is still used today by Caribbean peoples and many

others as a blood purifier. Because it contains several phytos-
terols, this herb is widely regarded as a tonic for the sex
glands and an aphrodisiac. It is also widely used to combat
arthritis and other bodily pains. Sarsaparilla is also recommended for digestive disorders, for skin diseases such as ringworm, as an eye wash, and, when taken on an empty stomach,
as a antidote against strong poisons. Sarsaparilla stimulates
the excretion of excess uric acid from the body and has long
been regarded as an aid to longevity. It is available in capsules
and tinctures.

Sassafras (*Sassafras officinalis*)—this herb was the chief
"medicine plant" for North American Indians long before the
white man appeared in North America. They prepared a tea
from the root and used it both as an everyday beverage and
to treat rheumatism. It was also used as a tonic after childbirth, as a tonic for stomach and bowels, as a blood purifier,
and as a remedy for bladder, kidney, and throat ailments.
Soups were flavored with a yellow powder made from the
dried leaves. The early colonists soon began using sassafras
as a tonic taken in springtime and to heal sore throats and
colds. The bark of the root has been scientifically proven to
contain antiseptic agents. The tea is still popular as a delicious
hot or cold tonic beverage, and a tea made from the bark
combats colds. It is also available in capsules and tinctures.

Slippery elm or Elm bark (*Ulmus fulva*)—this versatile
and soothing herb has many uses, both internal and external.
It is one of the best soothers of irritated digestive and respiratory tracts. Slippery elm can be purchased at drug stores
and health food stores in either the stick, chip, powder, or
capsule form.

Thyme (*Thymus serpyllum*)—this common culinary herb
has a long history of medical use, mainly because the thymol
it contains is a proven antiseptic. It disinfects, cleanses, and
purifies, and can be found in soaps (Pears), shampoos, bath
oils, mouthwashes, and chemical-free household cleansers.
Thyme tea alleviates coughing, sluggish digestion, and the
pain of uterine disorders. Studies suggest that thyme may protect the DNA from free radicals. Do not use for more than
one week as excessive use can lead to symptoms of poisoning

and overstimulation of the thyroid gland. Thyme is available loose and dried and in capsules.

Uva ursi (*Arctostaphyllos uva ursi*)—also known as bear berry, this indigenous herb is a staple in kidney and bladder remedies because of its diuretic properties and its remarkable ability to heal bladder infections. It is available loose and dried, in capsules and tinctures.

Valerian root (*Valeriana officinalis*)—a top-selling herb in Europe, valerian root is catching on quickly in the United States for its efficacy in promoting sleep and relaxation without the side effects of pharmaceutical sleep aids. Another advantage is that valerian root has no synergistic reaction with alcohol, which means that, unlike pharmaceutical sleeping pills, valerian will not produce an exaggerated and potentially dangerous effect when combined with alcohol. Valerian does cause allergic reactions in some people, so try a small amount at first. It is available in teas, capsules, and tinctures.

White clover—similar in many ways to red clover but less powerful, white clover is unique in its ability to ward off the mumps. If the tea or the blossoms are not available, eat white clover honey instead.

Wood betony (*Betonic officinalis*)—the ancient Greeks listed this plant as a remedy for no less than forty-seven diseases, particularly for digestive disorders, nervous diseases, prolonged infections, coughing, and chronic inflammation of the bladder and kidneys. It is available in capsules and tinctures.

How to Make
Your Own Herbal Remedies

Herbs packaged in tea bags tend to have lost much of their beneficial properties. It's best to gather the fresh herb yourself and use it immediately, whenever possible. If you buy dried herbs or dry them yourself, store them in tightly sealed containers to preserve their freshness. Always use pure water and organic ingredients in making your remedies. Do not use aluminum wares for making any herbal preparations. Preparations made in aluminum utensils can cause stomach ulcers. Enamel, glass, and stainless steel pots are best.

• *Basic Tea (Infusion) Recipe*
An infusion is a tea made from an herb, usually the leaves, flowers, and some berries. Bring pure water to a boil. The standard formula for an infusion is one teaspoon of dried herb to one cup of boiling water, although you might use less herb if the herb is very strong, more if it is weak. If you are using green (fresh) herbs, use one-half ounce of herb to one pint of boiling water. Remember: never boil the herb *with* the water, as boiling can make the herb lose its medicinal properties, unless you are preparing seeds, barks, roots, branches, and some leaves and berries (see Decoction, below). With most flowers and leaves, pour the boiling water *over* the herb. Then steep in a covered container for five to ten minutes. Strain and drink while warm. (If you prefer a sweeter-tasting tea, add one-half teaspoon of either cardamom powder or licorice root powder to the herb and steep together. You won't need to do this with fennel, which is naturally sweet.)

- *Decoction*

A decoction is also a tea, but it's stronger, and it is actually boiled or simmered. This is the method used to extract the mineral salts and bitter principles—the medicinal properties—from barks, roots, branches, and some leaves and berries. Use one teaspoon of herb to one cup of water. Boil for ten to thirty minutes. The longer you boil, the more medicinal properties you extract, but how long you boil also depends on the herbal materials you are using. Strain out the boiled plant parts before drinking.

- *Tinctures*

Chop the herb finely and add one ounce of herb to one pint of lab-proof alcohol (*not* rubbing alcohol!) or vodka. Shake daily. After two weeks, strain, and use according to instructions. The usual dose is one teaspoonful in one-half cup of warm water, three times a day.

- *Liniment*

Use the herb and isopropyl alcohol in the same proportions as a tincture. *For external use only.*

- *Balm or Salve*

Use either fresh or dried herbs and chop up very finely. For balms, salves, and poultices, the formula is usually one part herb to four parts of whatever you mix it with. Cook in pure, cold-pressed olive oil or another cold-pressed vegetable oil over a very low flame in a double boiler. Do not use iron pots because they contain tannic acid. Use only stainless steel, glass, or porcelain. Do not boil the herb. Cook for ten to thirty minutes, depending on the herb. Once the herb properties are extracted, strain off the roughage, then add slowly either cocoa butter or lanolin or beeswax until the desired consistency is reached. As the mixture cools, it hardens. *For external or topical use only.*

- *Baths*

Bathing and the proper care of the skin are far more important to the health of the body than many people realize. Somehow the skin is not generally thought of as a vital organ such as the heart, liver, or lungs. Yet science tells us that if the skin fails to function even for a few hours, all the internal organs can break down. The nervous system can become paralyzed and the kidneys, liver, and heart can become toxic to the point of failure.

The skin performs many essential functions. Its pores allow the body to eliminate wastes, more than the lungs, bowels, and kidneys combined. The skin regulates body temperature, conserving heat when outside temperatures are cold and perspiring when the body becomes overheated. In severe scaldings or third-degree burns where two-thirds of the skin is destroyed, death follows shortly—the result of the reflex destruction of the internal organs. Likewise, if the skin is completely coated or covered with a substance through which no air can penetrate, an individual will soon die. He becomes poisoned by his own gases and toxins, and the increased internal temperature causes inflammation of the visceral organs. Cases are recorded in which individuals have died in a very short time after their bodies were covered with impervious material such as paint.

The ancients recognized the value of bathing in promoting the skin's optimum functioning. Magnificent buildings were erected to serve as public baths, and herbs were added to the baths for esthetic and medicinal purposes. Hydrotherapy is still very popular in European countries, and you can have your own herbal bath in the privacy of your bathroom. To prepare an herbal bath, use either of the following methods:

1. Cover the herbs to be used with boiling water, lower the heat, cover, and allow to simmer for ten to fifteen minutes. Strain the decoction and add to the bath water or use it as a final rinse.

2. Add an equal amount of borax to the fresh or dried herbs being used to soften the water. (Borax crystals are optional.) Place the mixture in a nylon, cloth or cheesecloth bag or a clean nylon stocking. Tie and hang on your hot water tap and fill the tub high enough so you can sit and soak for ten to fifteen minutes. Or you can simply drop the bag into the bath water. Because the skin absorbs so much, it's a good idea to always

include a healing herb whenever you do take a bath. The water temperature should be warm, neither too hot nor too cold, either of which can be debilitating. A warm bath soothes, rather than shocks, the body. Aromatic oils can also be used, placed directly in the bath water with baking soda added to disperse the oil.

• *Clays*

Herbs mixed in healing clays are wonderful external applications that naturally extract boils, cysts, and tumors.

• *Poultices*

A poultice is used to draw impurities from the body by applying it externally with moist heat. Bruise or crush the medicinal parts of the plant to a pulpy mass and heat. If you are using dry herbs, mix with hot cornmeal to make a poultice and apply to affected area. Aloe gel is also effective for this purpose. Or you can grind up an herb and mix it with pure cold-pressed vegetable oil or water to make a paste. Another alternative is to simply take whatever is strained off when you are making an infusion or decoction, and use that as the base for a poultice. Or you can dip a clean cloth in the tea or decoction and apply it to the affected area. Ginger compresses are an example of a popular poultice used to bring heat and circulation to an area and to break up congestion. Soak a washcloth in very hot ginger water and apply to the affected area until the heat fades.

• *Aromatic Waters*

Pure water blended with fragrant herbs and flowers such as lavender and rose make aromatic waters. They can be used as skin toners, tonics and body washes or hair rinses. Never use chlorinated or fluoridated water when making aromatic waters. Use instead pure spring water, rain water, or distilled water. Prepare the waters in ceramic or glass containers. Use one cup of dried herb to one pint of pure water in a quart jar with a tight-fitting lid. Put in a convenient place and shake once or twice a day for two weeks. Strain and store in small glass vials with tight-fitting lids.

• *Capsules*

Almost any herb can be powdered and placed in a gelatin capsule. The standard capsule size is referred to as ''00.''

Capsules allow you convenience and mobility. You can swallow them with water, and you still have the option of opening the capsules, pouring out the contents, and adding hot water for tea or making pastes for a poultice.

• *Holistic Healing*

A basic premise followed by most herbal healers is that even if a condition seems to affect one organ only, you must treat the entire person. Another tenet of herbology is that different herbs are best used during specific times of the year. Roots and barks are considered most appropriate for use in wintertime, while leaves and flowers are best used during summertime. Spicy herbs such as cayenne promote resistence to infection and stimulate circulation. Dry herbs should not be used after one year, as they lose fifty percent of their effectiveness, even if you picked and dried them yourself. Roots, barks and some berries can be kept and used longer than most leaves. Herbs can be divided into several basic groups. *Tonic* herbs regenerate the digestive system, reviving energy and stimulating function. Because they are used to start an action, they should be taken for the short term only, as after prolonged use they can leach out essential vitamins and minerals. A good example of a tonic herb is goldenseal root, which regenerates mucus membranes anyplace in the body. Its bitter properties stimulate the functions of the gall bladder, liver, and salivary glands. However, if overused, those secretions can cause irritation in the mucus membrane. *Nutritive* herbs soothe, calm, and build, and can therefore be used for long periods. A good example of an herb with powerful healing properties is yarrow leaf or flower. *Carminative* herbs expel gas, stimulate stomach secretions, and help the stomach to absorb and assimilate nutrients. A good example is spearmint, an herb more soothing to the digestive system than peppermint, yet equally effective as a carminative. *Astringent* and *disinfectant* herbs cleanse, eliminate, and break down excess matter, such as as the excess mucus created by an ulcerated area. Raspberry leaf is a good example of a soothing, easy-to-take astringent herb.

Herbs for the nervous system are as follows: *Nervines* build the central nervous system (brain), the peripheral system (spine), and the nerves that correspond to organ systems. *Antispasmodics* relax and regulate nerve function in both the autonomic and voluntary systems. They help relieve cramps, spasms, tension headaches, aching knees, and spinal pain. *Cephalics* are usually flowers and work specifically on the brain to help you relax.

Unless otherwise indicated, herbs should be taken at least one-half hour before meals or at least two hours after them.

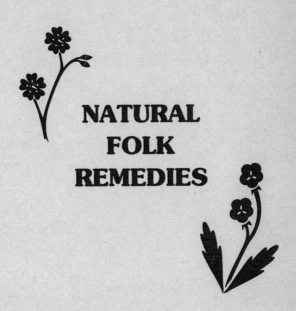

NATURAL
FOLK
REMEDIES

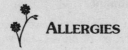

ALLERGIES

Peppermint Steam

When allergic reaction causes the mucus in your sinuses to dry up, this steam is a great reliever. Pour one quart of boiling water into a bowl containing one-quarter ounce of peppermint leaves. You can also use two or three drops of peppermint essential oil, which is more concentrated. Make a tent of a towel and breathe the steam for ten to fifteen minutes, inhaling deeply through your nose.

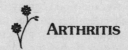

ARTHRITIS

Increasingly, the role of allergic reactions is being explored as a major cause of some forms of arthritis. These allergies can be to food, chemicals, or other substances in the environment. It is a good idea to find out what may be causing an arthritic reaction. You can do this by listing all foods you crave or eat regularly and the substances with which you come into regular contact. Eliminate those foods or substances, one at a time, for three or four days. Then reintroduce them, one by one, into your diet and/or immediate surroundings. If symptoms flare up after reintroducing a particular food or substance, that item is likely to be a culprit. The process of elimination and gradual reintroduction can be used to target any suspected allergen.

The following folk remedies help by relieving arthritic pain.

Combination Liniment

Combine one ounce each of sunflower seed oil, oil of turpentine, oil of camphor, oil of cloves, and wintergreen oil. This powerful liniment helps alleviate the discomfort of rheumatism and arthritis.

Sassafras Combination Arthritis Remedy

This traditional remedy works best during the earlier stages of the disease and should be taken over a long period of time.

Combine one ounce each of prickly ash bark, sassafras bark, and wood betony herb. Boil the barks only at a low, rolling boil in three pints of water for twenty to thirty minutes. Pour the hot liquid over the wood betony. Allow to cool, then strain. Take one-half cup, three to four times a day. If you add one-quarter teaspoon of ground ginger root and honey to taste, this beverage also remedies the sleeplessness that often accompanies the pain of arthritis.

Dandelion Tea

Brew a tea from the fresh leaves, if possible (using the basic tea recipe). Drink one cup, three or four times a day. This remedy, as well as the following, help treat arthritis by purifying the liver.

Cherries

Cherries are rich in vitamin C, so eat as much as you want of these delicious fruits to help reduce arthritic inflammation.

Gooseberries

These berries are said to prevent arthritis and many liver disorders. Eat freely.

Grape Fast

Grape fasts, usually lasting three or four days, are old and popular remedies said to help cure arthritis and rheumatism by eliminating toxins from the body and by aiding in the repair of damaged heart muscles. If you decide to try a grape fast, you must consult your doctor first.

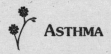

ASTHMA

Do not use any alternative asthma cures without checking with your doctor!

Honeysuckle

The blossoms and leaves of this deliciously fragrant flower are beneficial to asthma and other respiratory complaints. They help soothe irritated mucus membranes and expel excess mucus. Eat fresh, raw honeysuckle, bruising and shredding the leaves and blossoms and mixing them with honey. Or make a tea from fresh or dried blossoms, using two teaspoons of honeysuckle to one cup of water. Brew for five to ten minutes. Take one cup, three times a day.

Red Clover Tea

This old Indian remedy, made from the blossoms (using the basic tea recipe), relieves asthma, as well as hoarseness, colds, coughs, and other respiratory irritation. Add honey and a squeeze of lemon. Sip hot, every hour or two.

Cherry Stem Syrup

This remedy is effective against asthma, bronchitis, as a fever reducer, and as a diuretic for the kidneys.

Prepare a decoction (using the basic decoction recipe) with

cherry stems and water. Cool, then strain, and add enough honey to make a syrup. Take by the teaspoonful, as needed.

Lemon Juice

Pure lemon juice, taken in generous quantities, helps relieve the symptoms of asthma. Avoid if you suffer from an over-acid stomach.

Cranberry Drink

Simmer one ounce of crushed cranberries in one quart of water till it reduces to a thick drink. Do not sweeten. This old American Indian remedy helps relieve asthma attacks, reduces fevers, and fights bladder infections.

Onion-Garlic Asthma Remedy

Combine one-half chopped onion, two chopped garlic cloves, and one pint of Irish moss jelly (you can purchase this sea-weed at Caribbean-American stores and in health food stores). Simmer for one-half hour. Cool and then strain the mixture through a sieve. Add one-half cup of honey to one pint of the mixture. Take one tablespoon every two hours, sipping slowly. Alternate with honey mixed with water and fresh lemon juice.

American Indian Honey-Egg Asthma Remedy

Place a whole egg in a cup and cover halfway with lemon juice. Leave for twelve hours so that the shell softens. Remove the egg, shell it, and beat the yolk and white together. Add the reserved lemon juice and use an equal amount of honey. Bring the mixture to a boil. When it begins to thicken, remove from stove. Cool and bottle. Take one teaspoon, two times a day, in the morning and at night.

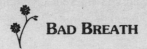

BAD BREATH

The most basic approach to keeping your breath fresh is to practice good oral hygiene, using proper brushing technique followed by flossing. It is also essential to brush your tongue. Check with your dentist to make sure your problem isn't caused by a festering tooth or gum disease. Eating yogurt or acidophilus culture may help bad breath by restoring the proper balance of bacteria to your intestinal tract. So might successful treatment of other causes of chronic indigestion. But gargling morning and night with any of the following teas will yield effective results.

Rosemary Tea Gargle

Brewed according to the basic tea recipe, this gargle is a tried-and-true method dating back several centuries. For extra protection, add either cloves or cinnamon. Also effective: gargling with fenugreek or peppermint teas.

Rosemary Wine

Boil a few handfuls of rosemary flowers in one pint wine for fifteen minutes. Cool, bottle, and sip a few mouthfuls to sweeten your breath.

Violet Mouthwash

Make a tea (using the basic tea recipe) with the flowers and top shoots of fresh violets. This healthy mouthwash keeps your breath fresh and sweet.

Seeds

Nibbling on cardomom seed or anise seed or a small piece of star of anise instead of an after-dinner mint is a great way to sweeten your breath and aid your digestion. Also effective: munching on parsley sprigs.

Charcoal Tablets

Take five tablets of purified charcoal to cleanse the intestinal tract and relieve flatulence and bad breath. Do not do this more than occasionally as charcoal could be carcinogenic.

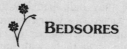 **BEDSORES**

Sugar and Honey

Pack regular granulated sugar (which has antibacterial properties) on the sores and cover with a thick, tight dressing. The sugar irritates the sore which, in turn, stimulates healing. In addition, sugar's acidity dilates the blood vessels, drawing more blood and lymph to the injury. Pure honey is equally effective.

Sugar–Egg White Amish Cure

Mix equal parts white sugar and an unbeaten egg white. Apply to the bedsore. Or you can combine one teaspoon of white sugar with a mix of equal parts of milk of magnesia and hydrogen peroxide, using just enough to make a thick paste. Apply to sore.

Fenugreek Seed Compress

This compress not only helps heal bedsores, but it is equally effective in treating wounds, cuts, boils, and external ulcerations.

Moisten the seeds slightly, then grind them into a thick paste, either with the blender or a mortar and pestle. Spread a thick layer on a clean piece of cloth or gauze and attach

securely to the boil. Change the dressing as the boil draws
and empties.

BLADDER AND KIDNEY AILMENTS

Your kidneys, along with your liver, are among the front-line
protection that filter out toxins entering your bloodstream.
The bladder and kidneys are relatively easily treated and
should be kept as healthy as possible. In New England, honey
and apple cider vinegar are taken regularly to keep the kidneys flushed. Pure cranberry juice, one cup taken three times
a day, and lemonade, taken whenever desired, are also considered stimulating tonics for the kidneys.

Approximately one out of every four women will experience the discomfort of a bladder infection at least once in her
lifetime. Most bladder infections are due to E. coli, a bacteria
normally present in the colon, so keeping that area clean is a
good preventative measure. It is always preferable to cure a
bladder infection by natural means, rather than by using antibiotics. This is because antibiotics tend to kill off ''good''
as well as ''bad'' bacteria, thereby upsetting the normal
balance. When the ecology of the urinary tract is upset, the
likelihood of another bladder infection increases sharply.
However, if the infection persists, antibiotics may be necessary. If you suffer from frequent urinary tract infections, see
a doctor in order to discover the underlying cause, which can
be anything from candidiasis to allergies.

During a bladder infection, it's best to drink distilled water
only. Avoid coffee, black tea, and alcohol. Take plenty of
vitamin C and rest.

Kidney Flush

Horseradish is a powerful herbal diuretic. It can be eaten by
itself, served with bread or fish, or mixed with vinegar or
diluted almost any way you can think of. The following is an

effective recipe to help the kidneys eliminate excess water.

Combine one ounce fresh, chopped horseradish with one-half ounce bruised mustard seed and one pint of boiling water. Steep in a covered pot for four hours, then strain. Take three tablespoons, three times a day. Or you can combine the horseradish with vegetable juice.

Asparagus Decoction

This is a great tonic for the urinary tract.

Wash two dozen asparagus stalks and cover with one quart of water. Bring to a boil, lower the heat, and simmer until the liquid is reduced by half. Cool, strain, and take one tablespoon every four hours.

Strawberry Prevention

Eat strawberries freely to help prevent the formation of kidney stones.

Onion Bladder Toner

Eaten cooked or raw, onions tone the bladder sphincter muscle and thus counter urinary incontinence.

Blueberries

Simply eating a few ounces of blueberries every night for a week or so when you have a kidney or bladder infection reduces your susceptibility to future infections.

Cranberry Juice

Nonsweetened, pure cranberry juice creates an environment that is hostile to infection-causing bacteria. Try to drink one quart a day. It is believed that cranberry juice contains a compound which our bodies convert into a substance that has an antibiotic effect on the urinary tract as it is excreted in the urine. Do not overuse, as even cranberry juice can throw off the body's natural balance. Drink plenty of distilled water to help remove excess acid and built-up minerals, especially if you have a history of kidney stones.

Cornsilk Tea

The "hair" of Indian corn or maize, which is usually discarded with the outer covering, is a great soothing herb and an effective diuretic for the treatment of bladder and kidney problems. Pour one pint of boiling water over two ounces of cornsilk. Steep for five to ten minutes. Take one-half cup every two or three hours. The fluid extract is also excellent.

Bladder Tea

Combine the following herbs:

> 1 tablespoon yarrow flowers and leaves
> 1 tablespoon uva ursi
> 1½ teaspoons juniper berry

Boil three cups of water and add one tablespoon of echinacea root. Simmer for twenty minutes, then pour over the combined herbs. Cover and steep for fifteen minutes. Drink one cup, three or four times a day. Juniper berry also tonifies the adrenals, but it should be used only at the beginning of an infection and avoided by those whose urinary tracts are constantly irritated. Uva ursi can be taken alone. It has antibiotic properties, and its active ingredient, arbutin, does not break down until it hits the urinary tract, where it gets to work. You can also combine tinctures of the above herbs, mixing them together in the same proportions. Take twenty drops in water, three to four times a day.

Goldenseal

During the first few days of a bladder infection or when you feel signs of an infection coming on, take two capsules of goldenseal root three times a day.

Marshmallow Root

Taken in a basic tea or in capsule form, one cup or one capsule, three times a day, this herb has a high mineral content and is wonderfully soothing for the urinary tract.

Burdock and Dandelion Root

Taken in tea or capsule form, one cup or capsule, three times a day, either of these roots is a great food for the bladder. They help to build up the urinary tract and stimulate its function.

Garlic

Taken raw, as a tea, or in a capsule, garlic acts as a powerful stimulant with diuretic, disinfectant and antiseptic, and antimucus action. Never take it alone, because of its irritating properties. Cooking tends to destroy garlic's medicinal properties. You can also take garlic in supplemental form.

Parsley Leaf Tea

Good food for the urinary tract, parsley root is high in minerals, breaks up stones, soothes, and acts as a powerful diuretic. Take in tea form. Steep two bunches of parsley in one gallon of boiling water for ten minutes. Sip as needed. (Parsley water, applied as a wash, is said to remove freckles!)

Kidney Stone Gypsy Drink

Heat one-half cup each of milk and wine. Skim off the curd and add a handful of chamomile flowers. Cover and let stand on a hot stove—but not on the burner—until the flowers dissolve. Drink as needed.

Watermelon Bladder Cure

Eat the meat of the watermelon, then slice the rind, boil it for twenty minutes, and drink it as a tea to help expel water from the body. Do not drink at bedtime because it is a strong diuretic. You can also buy dried watermelon pills in Chinese stores.

Flaxseed-Lemon Kidney Tonic

Combine four tablespoons flaxseed with one quart of water. Bring to a boil, then simmer for ten minutes. Add the fresh juice of one lemon. Add enough water to make a tea. Drink one-half cup every two hours, as needed.

Apple-Honey Kidney Tonic

Slice, but do not peel, four apples and place on a cookie sheet lined with wax or brown paper. Dry in a low oven with the door open. When the apples are dried, close the oven door and bake until the slices are completely browned. To make the tea, pour one pint of boiling water over three or four slices. Cover and steep for ten minutes. Add honey to taste. Drink as needed.

Fenugreek Tea Kidney and Bladder Cleanse

When mucus linings become irritated, they automatically secrete excess mucus as a protective measure. This excess mucus can trap toxins, then harden and impede the full functioning of the related organ. Fenugreek seed tea helps the urinary tract rid itself of that excess mucus and the toxins it holds.

Pour one cup of boiling water over two teaspoons of fenugreek seeds. Steep for five to ten minutes, then strain. Drink one cup three or four times a day.

Kidney Root Tonic

Combine one ounce each asparagus root, celery root, fennel, and parsley root and place in a jar. Pour in one pint of boiling water and steep overnight. Strain and take one-half cup of the liquid with a few drops of fresh lemon juice before meals, for two or three days in a row. Repeat this treatment every few months to keep your kidneys flushed and toned.

Kidney Toning Tea

Combine the following herbs:

> 4 tablespoons dandelion root
> 4 tablespoons parsley root
> 2 tablespoons marshmallow root
> 1 tablespoon ginger root

Make a decoction (using the basic decoction recipe). Strain. Take one cup, three times a day.

BLOAT

If bloat is a chronic problem, see your doctor to determine and correct the underlying cause. But if this happens only occasionally, here is what you can try.

Onion Juice

Boil four onions in a quart of water. Drink the water freely to reduce retention of fluids.

Indian Seed Teas

Excess fluid that is accumulated in the body can be flushed out of the system with a tea made from any one of the following seeds: anise, caraway, or fennel. Use one teaspoon of seeds to one cup of boiling water. Simmer for twenty to thirty minutes. Strain and sip slowly while still warm. Tea made from anise is also excellent for expelling gas in the intestinal tract and to quiet persistent, dry coughs.

Pears

Eat this fruit freely to help the body eliminate excess fluid.

Dandelion Leaves

Taken raw in a salad, lightly steamed as a vegetable, or made into a tea (using dried or fresh leaves according to the basic tea recipe), this highly nutritious green is an effective diuretic and a stimulant to almost every internal organ.

Dandelion-Juniper Tea

Make a decoction (using the basic decoction recipe) with one-half ounce each of dandelion root and juniper berries and one quart of water. Bring to a boil, cover, and simmer until the liquid is reduced to a pint. Take one cup every four hours.

Parsley Tea

Place one bunch of parsley in one quart of boiling water. Simmer for twenty minutes. Strain and drink as needed.

Parsley Milk

Combine two pounds of fresh, chopped parsley with one quart of milk. Place in pan and bake in your oven at 300 degrees until the liquid reduces to one pint. Cool and strain. Take one tablespoon every two hours for no more than three days in a row.

Asparagus

Steamed asparagus is a diuretic, as is the water it is steamed in.

Irish-American Potato Cure

Wash one handful of potato peelings and place in pot. Cover with water, bring to a boil, cover, and simmer for twenty minutes. Strain and take two tablespoons in one cup of water, three to four times a day.

Watermelon Seed Tea

Brew this tea using the basic decoction recipe with a handful of seeds to one quart of water. Drink one cup, three times a day.

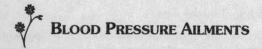 # BLOOD PRESSURE AILMENTS

See your doctor if overly high or low blood pressure is chronic. For high blood pressure, several recommendations are helpful. Cut down on salt and eat more fruits, grains, and vegetables. Add both onions and garlic to your daily diet in order to drop your blood pressure by as much as twenty points. Onions contain prostaglandin A, a hormonelike substance that can lower blood pressure. Garlic's effect on the blood and circulation system is more complex, but it is equally effective.

Stewed Celery

Cook a bunch of cleaned celery stalks in one gallon of water until the stalks are soft. Eat the vegetable and drink the water to reduce high blood pressure. Or you can brew a tea (using the basic decoction recipe) from celery seeds.

Potato Peel Decoction

This humble folk remedy helps reduces high blood pressure. Simmer five clean potatoes in one pint of water for twenty minutes. Cool and strain. Drink one cup, twice a day.

Pears

Eat this fruit freely to reduce high blood pressure.

Watermelon Seed Tea

Watermelon seeds contain cucurbocitrin, a substance that dilates capillaries, thereby reducing the burden placed on the larger blood vessels.

Brew this tea using the basic decoction recipe. Drink one cup three times a day to help relieve high blood pressure.

Cranberry Blood Pressure Reducer

Simmer crushed whole cranberries in enough water to cover until they are lightly cooked, softened but not reduced to a pulp. This New England remedy also purifies the blood and clears the complexion.

Huckleberry Root Tea

This is an old Canadian Indian recipe. Brew a tea with dried huckleberry roots (using the basic decoction recipe). Strain. Drink one cup, three times a day.

Nettle Tea

Nettles are rich in iron, which is essential to healthy circulation and normal blood pressure.

Brew a strong tea from the nettles (using the basic decoction recipe). Take one cup, three times a day to lower blood pressure.

Fig Blood Pressure Builder

Figs, fresh or dried, are rich in calcium, iron, and copper, all important to build blood. Figs also help correct overly low blood pressure.

Blood Pressure Regulating Tincture

Combine the following herb powders:

> 6 teaspoons hawthorn berries
> 3 teaspoons motherwort
> 3 teaspoons ginseng root
> 2 teaspoons ginger root

If you cannot get the herb powders, use the dried herbs and chop finely. Mix well. Make a tincture with a pint of brandy (using the basic tincture recipe). Cap well and shake a few times a day for fourteen days. Strain out the herbs.

Take one teaspoon of the tincture with one tablespoon of wheat germ oil, three times a day.

Dandelion Tea

Brew a strong tea from the leaves (doubling the amount of dandelion to water given in the basic tea recipe). This tea contains many blood-purifying nutritive salts and it is also believed by the Gypsies to normalize blood pressure.

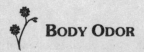 **BODY ODOR**

If you practice good hygiene and body odor persists, see your doctor. The offensive odor may be indicative of an underlying health problem.

Underarm Sweetener

For a safe and effective deodorizer, splash white vinegar under your arms or dust them with baking soda. You can also add one-half cup of baking soda to your hot bath water.

Amish Deodorant

Heat a small pan on the stove into which you mix well one tablespoon of cold-pressed vegetable oil, two tablespoons of corn starch, and two tablespoons of baking soda. Stir until thoroughly blended, then cool and store in a closed container in a cool, dark place. Apply as needed.

BOILS

A boil is an infection of a sweat gland or hair follicle. Traditional herbalism views boils as an indication of a body's low resistance to infection and internal impurities coming to the surface. They usually recommend drinking teas made from such herbs as echinacea, goldenseal, barberry, yellow dock, red clover, nettle, sassafras, and cayenne (prepared according to the basic tea recipe). Another recommendation is to chew burdock seeds or drink the tea to cleanse an overburdened liver of toxins. Do not squeeze boils. Use hot compresses instead to allow the pus to empty out on it own. Even plain hot water is effective, but poultices are even better. Keep the surrounding area free from infection by painting it with iodine and washing your hands and the surrounding area with germicidal soap.

Boil Hot Soak

If the boil is on a part of your body that's easily immersible in water, simply use a basin of water heated to a temperature as hot as you can stand and soak as long as possible.

Hot Bottle Remedy

Fill a small-mouth jar with boiling water. Let stand a few
minutes to heat the jar. Pour out the water and immediately
hold the mouth of the jar to the boil. As it cools, the jar will
create a suction action that draws out the boil.

Onion Poultice

Pound an onion with a mallet to make a poultice that is
equally effective for boils, ulcers, abscesses, and insect stings!
Cover, secure, and leave on overnight.

A variation calls for roasting the onion. Cut it in half and
apply while warm to the infected area. Cover, secure, and
leave on overnight. Save the other half for the second application.

Amish Raw Egg Compress

Take the thin membranelike skin found on the inside of a
freshly broken egg shell and lay it on the boil.

American Indian Herbal Poultices

Crush any of the following herbs: violet leaves, wild pansy
leaves, catnip leaves, yarrow, wild dock leaves, or ground
flaxseed. Heat and apply to the boil while they're warm.
Cover and secure well. You can also steam those leaves
lightly and apply to the boil.

Raw Carrot Poultice

Shred carrots and add vitamin E or wheat germ oil from a
freshly pricked capsule. Apply to infected area, cover with
gauze and leave on overnight.

Cranberry Poultice

Crush whole fresh cranberries into a mash. Apply in a thick coat to a clean piece of cloth. Cover the boil and secure well. Leave on overnight. This old American Indian remedy also works well on fever blisters.

Lemon Poultice

Heat a thick slice of lemon and apply to infected area. Cover and leave on overnight.

Old Testament Fig Poultice

This remedy comes straight from Isaiah in the Old Testament, which describes the King of Judah, Hezekiah's, cure for boils. Roast a fig. Split and apply to the boil. Or you can split the fig and then soak it for a few minutes in warm water. Apply to the boil. Cover with a bandage and secure. Leave on overnight and in the morning, the boil should be gone!

Honey and Fig Poultice

Slice a ripe fig in half. Dip the cut side in good-quality honey. Place against boil, cover, and secure. Leave on constantly, changing the poultice two or three times a day, until the drawing action has stopped.

Slippery Elm Poultice

Make a compress by mixing slippery elm powder with hot water or a cold-pressed vegetable oil. Place on boil, tape in place, and leave on overnight.

Banana Compress

Apply the inside of a banana skin to the boil. Cover and tape securely. Leave on overnight.

Cabbage Compress

Chop cabbage leaves and place directly on boil. Cover and tape in place. Leave on as long as you desire.

Comfrey Compress

Make a tea several times more concentrated than the basic tea recipe using comfrey roots or leaves. Dip a clean cloth or gauze into the tea and tape onto the boil.

Flaxseed Compress

Make a strong tea with flaxseed, then dip a clean cloth or gauze into the hot solution and apply to the boil. Do this frequently, every three to four hours.

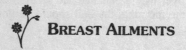 **BREAST AILMENTS**

Breast Milk Increaser

Nettle tea (using the basic tea recipe), one cup, three to four times a day, increases milk flow and quantity.

Baby Weaner

Sage tea (using the basic tea recipe), one cup, three or four times a day, dries up breast milk when you are weaning your child.

Breast Soreness

Roast lightly bruised papaya leaves and rub on breasts to relieve the soreness caused by nursing.

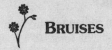

BRUISES

If you bruise easily, it may mean your capillaries are weak and damage easily, a sign of vitamin C and/or bioflavenoid deficiency. Vitamin C and bioflavenoids, which are found in the peel and white skin under the peel of citrus fruits, strengthen the capillaries.

Lemon Water

This drink helps make up deficiencies in vitamin C and bioflavenoids. Wash and cut six lemons, including the peelings, into small pieces. Place in a pot with one and one-half quarts of water and bring to a boil. Turn off the heat. Cover and let stand until cool. Refrigerate, tightly covered, overnight. Drink one strained cup three times a day.

Witch Hazel Compresses

Distilled witch hazel, applied to the bruise with a clean cloth or cotton pad as often as desired, speeds healing.

Ice Cube Compress

The simplest and most effective way to reduce bruises, especially immediately after the injury, is simply to apply a cloth soaked in ice-cold water or just place ice cubes in a towel and secure to the bruised area. Leave on for about twenty minutes, take off for about three minutes, then on again, repeating this process for several hours.

Hypertonic Cure

Mix one pint of hot water with one tablespoon of sea salt or Epsom salts, one teaspoon of baking soda, and one teaspoon of boric acid. Apply either as a hot compress or as a soak.

Huckleberry Poultice

This North American Indian remedy works on bruises as well as cuts. Crush enough huckleberries to make a poultice that will cover the affected area. Spread on a clean cloth or piece of gauze and cover the bruise. Secure and leave on overnight.

Papaya Juice

Apply the juice directly to bruises or soak a clean piece of gauze or cloth in the juice and then apply to affected area.

 BURNS

Cold water and ice provide instant relief, but for relief plus speedier healing, try any of the following.

Ice Water-Lavender Reliever

Place the burned area in ice water for ten minutes or longer. Dry and apply two drops of lavender oil.

Aloe Vera

The leaves of this succulent provide a healing ointment. Cut a piece from a lower leaf of a plant over five years old and apply the gel that oozes out to the burn. Or slice the leaf lengthwise and apply the inside to the burn. If you do not have a plant or your plant is not old enough, you can buy the gel—not the juice—in a bottle or tube at your local health food store.

Honey

Pure, natural honey, applied under a dry dressing every two or three hours promotes the healing of burns (and ulcers).

Yogurt

Apply the yogurt—only the pure, natural brands, not the supermarket variety which contains refined starches—several times to prevent it from drying out.

Vitamin E

Pierce vitamin E capsules and apply to burn. Do not use vitamin E from the bottle as your hands might contaminate the contents.

Vitamin E–Comfrey Ointment

Put one-half cup of vitamin E or wheat germ oil and one-half cup of honey in a blender and run at low speed until they are thoroughly mixed together. Add enough comfrey leaves to make a thick paste. Blend at medium speed until the mixture is smooth. Store in refrigerator to keep the oil from turning rancid. Apply as needed. The vitamin E and honey soothe the skin and also promote healing. This is also effective for sunburns.

Banana Skin Poultice

Apply the inside of a banana skin to the burned area. Cover and tape securely. Leave on overnight.

Onion and Salt

To draw out the heat from scalding burns, apply a piece of onion with a pinch of salt.

Slippery Elm Poultice

Mix the powdered bark of slippery elm with enough water to make a soft paste. Apply as a poultice to heal burns, ulcers, and skin diseases.

Burn Relieving Tea

This tea is meant to be taken internally to soothe the pain of a burn and aid in the healing process.

Mix together equal parts of the following herbs: red clover blossoms, nettles, skullcap, marshmallow. Simmer two ounces of the herb mixture in two pints of water for twenty to thirty minutes. Sip one-half cup every two hours, until the pain subsides.

Baking Soda Paste

Blend bicarbonate of soda with enough pure water to make a paste. Apply to burn. **Note**: For serious burns, it is important to feed the patient nutrient-packed foods—fresh vegetables and fruit, grains, legumes, and meats—up to 5,000 to 6,000 calories a day—to help the body in its repair work.

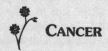

CANCER

Progress towards finding a cure for cancer through drugs and surgery has been snail-like, but discoveries concerning how you can prevent cancer by choosing to eat the right foods and avoiding others have been proceeding by leaps and bounds. The most recent studies suggest that better nutrition—which includes the use of herbal nutrients—is your best preventive weapon against cancer.

At the National Cancer Institute (NCI), a program to design cancer-fighting foods has been underway for several years and early findings are promising. We all know the tremendous risk factor of smoking. But other factors are emerging. Studies suggest that restricting dietary fat is essential and there are suspicions that meat, especially meat that has been cured in sodium nitrate or nitrite (hot dogs, sausages, smoked fish) or from animals raised on a diet of antibiotics and other chemicals, may help to determine who gets cancer.

Other cancer-prevention tips: cut down on caffeine and alcohol. Garlic and onions top the list of what you should eat. It is estimated that in China's Shandong province where people eat large amounts of garlic and onions cut their risk of stomach cancer by as much as 40 percent. A study of more than 41,000 women in Iowa showed that those who added garlic to their food at least once a week reduced their risk of colon cancer by 35 percent. Allium compounds, contained in both garlic and onions, increase levels of enzymes that break down potential carcinogens. Allium compounds may also increase the activity of cancer-fighting immune cells. Several other food ingredients could protect against a variety of cancers: flaxseed, mustard, burdock, kale, parsley, carrots, and rosemary. Figs are also said to contain anticancer factors that may prevent precancerous conditions from forming. The following are other food substances that have shown promising results in scientific studies.

Green and Black Tea

Tea leaves contain antioxidants called polyphenols, which can prevent damage to DNA. If cells do become cancerous, certain polyphenols seem to inhibit their growth and help the body rid itself of carcinogens more rapidly. Green tea contains antioxidants that may lessen the incidence of lung cancer among the Japanese, who are some of the heaviest smokers in the world. Skin tumor growth in laboratory animals is slowed when green tea is applied topically. One Chinese study showed that a group of tea drinkers cut their risk of cancer of the esophagus by more than half compared to non–tea drinkers. These results only apply to green or black teas, not herbal. Note: Be sure you do not drink the tea when it's too hot. Scientists estimate that your risk of esophagal cancer increases if you drink the beverage when it's boiling hot.

Licorice Root

Glycyrrhizin, the sweet substance in licorice, prevents the formation of a byproduct of testosterone that might stimulate the growth of prostate cancer, and it seems to protect the DNA.

Do not use licorice root if you suffer from high blood pressure.

Tomatoes

Tomatoes are loaded with vitamin C, a potent antioxidant that destroys DNA-destroying free radicals. Vitamin C is found in many vegetables and fruits, but tomatoes also contain lycopene, which may explain why a recent Italian study found that people who ate raw tomatoes at least seven times weekly cut their risk of several cancers in half, compared to those who ate tomatoes not more than once a week. Tomatoes are also rich in p-coumaric acid and chlorogenic acid, which attach to nitric oxides in the foods we eat and remove them from the body before they can form cancer-causing nitrosamines.

Beet Juice

Some German researchers reported effective results with leukemia and tumorous diseases in patients who drank the freshly expressed juice from two and one-half pounds of beets every day.

Oranges and Lemons

These citrus fruits raise levels of enzymes that break down carcinogens and stimulate cancer immunity. Citrus fruits also contain a substance that destroys carcinogens and removes them from the system. When rats in one study were exposed to a carcinogen and then drank their body's equivalent of a gallon of orange juice a day, they developed 40 percent fewer signs of cancer.

Grapes

Grapes contain large amounts of an acid that keeps the body from producing certain enzymes needed by cancer cells. In one study, mice were given an extract of Concord grapes that proved as effective as the cancer drug methotrexate in slowing tumor growth. Grapes are packed with other "helpful" chemicals that may inhibit the formation of blood clots, and a natural fungicide that slows down the accumulation of "bad" LDL cholesterol.

Chile and Cayenne Pepper

Researchers initially studied chile pepper under the assumption that it might cause cancer. But Mexicans have relatively few cases of stomach cancer, even though they eat a lot of chiles. The capsaicin in hot peppers may neutralize the carcinogenic effect of nitrosamines and keep the cancer-causing elements in cigarette smoke from attaching to DNA, thus preventing DNA damage that can lead to lung and other cancers.

Soybeans

Soy is rich in a chemical that fights cancer several ways. Cancer cells in the breast and ovaries are stimulated by estrogen. This chemical contained in soy mimics estrogen and fills up receptors for the actual hormone, thus lowering the body's estrogen level. Soy may also prevent small blood vessels from forming around cancer cells, so that they cannot receive oxygen and nutrients. A recent study of six women found that a soy-heavy diet lengthened the menstrual cycle by roughly two and a half days, reducing exposure to estrogen. That could explain why Japanese women, whose daily diet includes soybeans and soy products, have one-fifth the rate of breast cancer as Americans.

Broccoli and Cabbage

These vegetables contain a wealth of cancer-fighting substances. Some stimulate the production of enzymes that weaken carcinogens and flush them out of the body. Others affect estrogen metabolism, encouraging the body to produce forms of the hormone that don't promote breast cancer. In a 1991 study, twelve volunteers took an extract of broccoli and cabbage every day for a week. Tests at the week's end showed a fifty percent increase in blood levels of "good" estrogen.

Red Clover Tincture

The Amish claim to prevent most cancers with red clover blossom tincture (using the basic tincture recipe). Take ten to twenty drops every morning, before breakfast.

Pau d'Arco Tea

This tea made from the bark of a Latin American tree is said to have anticarcinogen properties. It is also highly recommended to fight the yeast infection known as *candida albicans*.

Boil for ten minutes, then steep for ten minutes more. Do not use packaged tea bags.

Fig Milk Poultice

This is another Amish remedy. Boil one pound of fresh figs in one gallon of fresh milk, until the figs soften. Remove them from the milk and stir until they turn into a paste. Apply a poultice to the skin cancer every twelve hours, cover and secure well.

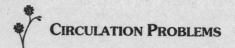 **CIRCULATION PROBLEMS**

Hawthorn Tea

Brew the leaves and flowers (using the basic tea recipe). Drink one cup, as needed.

Pine Oil Bath

Exercise is the best way to stimulate your circulation. If you suffer from cold hands and feet and you cannot exercise, a warm bath will do much to bring comfort to your entire body.

Add one tablespoon of pine oil to your bath water to stimulate circulation and refresh your system.

Marigold-Nettle Bath

Make a quart decoction of equal parts of marigold, nettle, and bladderwrack (using the basic tea recipe). Strain and add to your bath water.

Instant Foot Warmer

Put finely ground cayenne pepper in a box and use a powder puff to lightly powder your feet with the pepper. Put on your socks and you're ready to go. When traveling to cold climes, carry along gelatin capsules of cayenne pepper. Open a capsule, pour the contents into your hands, and rub the pepper into your feet. Be careful to wash your hands thoroughly with soap and water after applying the pepper because if transferred from your hands to your face, cayenne will irritate your eyes and mucous membranes.

You can also swallow one capsule of cayenne, twice a day, or eat the whole peppers to pep up circulation. Take plenty of water.

Red Pepper Soak

Soak your cold feet in a basin of hot water into which you've mixed a teaspoon or so of cayenne pepper.

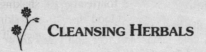

CLEANSING HERBALS

Free radicals are highly reactive atoms on molecules that can damage cells and cause genetic mutation. Scientists today attribute many diseases, as well as aging of the body, to the damage caused by free radicals. The notion of antioxidants, substances that fight chemically reactive free radicals in the body, seems a modern one, but natural healers have been using herbs for their antioxidant properties for thousands of years.

Milk Thistle and Ginkgo Biloba: Free Radical Destroyers

Pliny the Elder, the Roman naturalist, wrote about medicinal uses of milk thistle, which modern research indicates has strong antioxidant properties. It is particularly effective against free radicals because it has been proven to act in the liver, where poisonous chemicals are detoxified. Ginkgo biloba, the world's oldest tree species, also contains powerful antioxidant properties. Both milk thistle and gingko biloba are effective for this use only if taken in standardized capsule forms. Drinking either herb in tea form may not bring the desired results. In the case of both milk thistle and ginkgo, the recommended dose is one 40 mg. tablet, three times a day.

Sarsaparilla Decoction

The North American Indians considered this root to be one of their most valuable remedies and dug it up during the months of July and September. They made teas from sarsaparilla root, chopping it finely and using the basic decoction recipe, as well as tinctures. To make the tincture, fill a bottle halfway with the finely chopped root, then add equal parts of water and pure lab-proof alcohol, filling the bottle all the way up. Let the bottle stand for fourteen days, shaking well every day. For serious cases of blood disease and skin eruptions, take four to five tablespoons a day plus one-half pint of the tea at the same time.

Burdock Root or Seed Tea

Boil four cups of water. Add one tablespoon of burdock root or seed. Simmer for twenty minutes. This makes three cups, which you should drink daily. This is particularly helpful for cleansing the blood and encouraging the kidneys to eliminate toxins.

Dandelion Tea

Brew a tea from the fresh leaves, if possible (using the basic tea recipe). Drink one cup, three or four times a day, to cleanse toxins from the liver, gallbladder, spleen, bladder, and kidneys.

Mulberries

Chew the fresh berries to cleanse and tone the liver.

Burdock-Sarsaparilla Tincture

Make a tincture (using the basic tincture recipe), combining equal parts of burdock seeds and sarsaparilla. Take thirty to sixty drops, three to four times a day.

Blood Cleansing Capsules

This remedy is especially effective in cases of blood poisoning and external infections.

Combine the following powdered herbs:

2 tablespoons goldenseal
4 tablespoons chaparral
6 tablespoons echinacea

Mix well and fill 00-size gelatin capsules. Take four capsules every four hours. As the conditions improve, reduce intake to three times a day for seven days.

Cerassee Leaf Tea (Mormodica Charantia)

An extremely popular medicine with Caribbean people, the leaves from this creeping herb are made into a tea (using the basic tea recipe) and used for colds, as a laxative, and as a blood cleanser. Research is currently underway to evaluate its use against cancer. In Jamaica, it is only taken for nine days straight, only when necessary, as prolonged use can cause liver damage. A cerassee bath is excellent for skin eruptions and acne. This herb should not be taken by diabetics as it masks the sugar content in the blood and urine. When very hot, the tea can also be taken for toothaches and mouth infections.

Blueberry Blood Cleanser

Mix together equal amounts of blueberry leaves, thyme, watercress, and powdered sassafras bark. Pour one cup of boiling water over one teaspoon of the mixture and let steep for ten to fifteen minutes. Cover and cool, then strain. Take one cup, four times a day, with little food.

Blood Purifying Tincture

This blood purifying remedy is a wonderful aid in the treatment of cancer, drug addiction, inflammatory conditions, any type of skin infections, tooth infections, colds, flu, and any condition where toxicity is a factor.

Combine the following powdered herbs:

2 tablespoons echinacea   1 tablespoon ginseng
2 tablespoons chaparral   1 tablespoon goldenseal

1 tablespoon yellow dock   1 tablespoon ginger
1 tablespoon garlic   1 tablespoon licorice
1 tablespoon sarsaparilla   1 tablespoon poke root
1 tablespoon sassafras

Mix well and combine two ounces of herb mixture with one cup of lab-proof alcohol. Steep for several days, then strain. Take one teaspoon in one-half cup of warm water, three times a day.

Amish Blood Purifying Tea

Mix together the following herb powders:

> 4 teaspoons dandelion root
> 4 teaspoons burdock root and seeds
> 4 teaspoons red clover blossoms
> 1 teaspoon fennel seeds

Pour one cup of boiling water over two tablespoons of the herb mixture. Steep for ten minutes. Strain. Drink two tablespoons thirty minutes after each meal.

Liver Cleanse Tea

This formula is a good cleanser for hepatitis. Boil ten cups of water and add two tablespoons each of dandelion root, burdock root, and yellow dock root. Simmer for ten minutes, then add two tablespoons of nettle. Simmer for ten more minutes. Add two tablespoons each of red clover, alfalfa, and peppermint. Simmer for ten minutes. Drink five to six cups a day.

Rosemary Liver Stimulator

A turn-of-the-century physician who specialized in natural remedies recommended drinking rosemary tea (using the basic tea recipe) throughout the day to stimulate torpid livers and as a tonic during the fall and spring months.

Liver-Gallbladder Stimulator

Brew chamomile and dandelion teas (using the basic tea recipe). Mix one part chamomile to two parts dandelion tea, and add one-half teaspoon of fresh lemon juice. Take one cup, three times daily. This tea also perks up slightly sluggish kidney function.

Beet Juice

One cup a day of freshly expressed beet juice (made in a juicer or in a blender with enough water added to make a juice) is said to be tonic and cleansing for the liver.

A variation calls for three ounces each of beet and carrot juice, combined with two ounces of celery juice.

Limeade Liver Cleanse

Combine the juice of two or three freshly squeezed limes with one cup of water and add honey to taste. Drink as desired.

Irish-American Lettuce Liver Cleanse

Chop up a small head of lettuce and simmer it in a quart of water for twenty minutes. Strain and take two tablespoons per hour to cleanse the liver.

Liver-Gallbladder Cleanse

This remedy is said to expel gallstones and prevent their formation. Take nothing but one cup of apple juice and hot water, every two hours for one or two days. The next morning, drink one cup of apple juice chased by one-half cup of olive oil.

Super Liver-Gallbladder Cleanse

This is my favorite,—gentle but effective. Mince one clove of garlic, a piece of ginger root approximately one inch square, two tablespoons of parsley, and place in a blender. Add one tablespoon of olive oil, eight ounces of water, and eight ounces of either fresh orange juice or organic apple juice. Divide into thirds and drink one portion before each of your three daily meals. Regular enemas are a helpful adjunct to this cleansing. Follow this regime for two to three weeks.

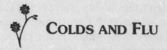 COLDS AND FLU

No other malady has inspired as many remedies—or defied our best efforts—as the common cold and flu. And most of the people of the world, no matter how far apart they may be in custom and distance, have relied on many of the same ingredients to combat these annoying—sometimes even life-threatening—ailments.

Any of these remedies will be more effective than antibiotics, which are generally useless against viruses—the culprits in colds and flus. These folk remedies are also more beneficial because they seek to bolster your body's own natural resistance while deploying natural antibiotic and antiviral properties.

Garlic is considered a potent natural antibiotic and blood purifier by many cultures of the world, including our own. It's best to use organic garlic, since it contains more antibiotic properties. The Russian medical establishment has harnessed garlic's antibiotic powers in the form of volatile oils or extracts called phitoncides, which are powerful natural germ killers. In most cases, the extracts are inhaled for prolonged periods. Other applications include local treatments on diseased tissues. Onions are equally healthful, and their use as a natural remedy dates back to the ancient Greeks and Romans. They are rich in vitamin C, which is proven by studies to have some effect in shortening the duration of a cold. Again, organic onions are recommended. Many other home remedies are based on liquids, which counter dehydration caused by vomiting or high fever, loosen congestion, and relieve sore throat and coughs. Hot liquids perform the same functions while also raising the temperature of the throat, which some people believe stops the reproduction of viruses. Cold and flu viruses often take hold first in the throat before spreading throughout the body.

Honey is another ingredient commonly found in cold and flu remedies. Its gooey texture is believed to coat sore throats and irritated membranes, soothing and protecting them. Recent theories claim that honey triggers the release of endorphins, the brain chemicals that relieve pain. It is certain, however, that honey does stimulate the production of saliva, thereby moistening the throat. Honey also has natural antibiotic properties, and it may also quiet a cough. But it should not be given to a child less than a year old because it can be contaminated with bacteria against which a child that young cannot defend itself.

Citrus fruits, another popular ingredient in home cures for colds and flu, are thought to establish an acidic environment in the throat in which viruses cannot flourish. Also, many fruits and vegetables contain high amounts of vitamins A and C, known to boost immunity.

Spices and spicy foods that contain chili pepper and cayenne are rich in capsaicin, the substance that sets your mouth on fire when you eat spicy food. Capsaicin causes tissues to release fluids and loosens mucus congestion.

Although few scientific confirm the claims made for the following cures, there is no end of persuasive anecdotal testimonials.

Classic Cold Cure

Preheat a double-size tea mug. Place two teaspoons of chamomile blossoms in the mug. Add the juice of one-half lemon, one tablespoon of honey, one-half teaspoon of ground cloves, one and one-half jiggers of brandy (not cognac) or dark rum. Add boiling water, fill to brim and allow to steep for at least four minutes. Strain. This remedy is best taken at the first signs of a cold.

Cold Killer

This remedy combines the four most powerful weapons against a cold. Mix together the following:

> 1 teaspoon cayenne pepper
> juice of one lemon
> 1 minced garlic clove
> 1 gram of Vitamin C (powdered)

The garlic and cayenne pepper have germicidal properties and make you sweat, which is always effective cold relief. The lemon contains vitamin C and bioflavenoids, which make the vitamin C work better.

Onion Juice

Fill a teacup with chopped onions, amd sprinkle with a tea-spoon of sugar. Place a saucer on top, then invert the cup so that it's upside down in the saucer. Place the cup and saucer in a warm place (stove top or warm oven) for several hours until the warm juice collects in the saucer. Spoon up onion juice and swallow. It tastes great and gets rid of whatever's ailing you.

Hot Toddy

Mix a shot of brandy and juice of one-half lemon into a tea cup. Pour in hot water and drink. Take enough of these and you'll forget you have a cold.

Onion Blender Cure

Dice one large onion (preferably red onion), add three pieces of garlic, and place in a blender with a tablespoon each of honey and lemon. Liquify until completely blended. You can either strain the mixture or pour it into a bottle. Swallow a teaspoonful every four hours. It actually tastes good!

Only for the Strong Garlic Cure

Chew one or two cloves of raw garlic, two or three times a day, until the cold seems to disappear, and for a few days after that. Cooking seems to lessen garlic's effectiveness, so take it raw. Or you can cut the clove into tiny pieces and swallow with water or put it in an empty 00-size gelatin capsule just before swallowing, otherwise the moisture will melt the capsule. If the taste or odor of garlic is offensive to you— or your closest companions—use one of the many fine brands of "deodorized" garlic pills or capsules on the market. Organic garlic is preferred as it has less potential allergens and more antibiotic properties.

Garlic and Lemon Tea

A delicious alternative to plain garlic, this tea is also enjoyed by children. Chop one clove of garlic into tiny pieces. Place in the bottom of a cup and press into a paste with a spoon. Add the juice of one-quarter small lemon. Put one teaspoon of peppermint or spearmint leaves in a pot, add the garlic-lemon mix, and pour in boiling water. Let steep for three to five minutes. Strain. Use honey is desired. Drink one cup, three times a day, until symptoms disappear and for two to three days after.

Garlic Milk Toddy

Heat a cup of milk until it's scalding hot. Add one tablespoon of honey and one teaspoon of butter. Stir until well mixed. Add one teaspoon of grated fresh garlic. Sip slowly one hour before bedtime.

Pickled Garlic Snacks

Many people object to chewing a garlic clove regardless of the health benefits. A more palatable way of enjoying garlic's benefits is to pickle it in miso and then eat it. Miso is a fermented soybean paste used in Asian cooking as a boullion and soup stock. The miso mellows the sharpness of the garlic and adds a salty yet slightly sweet flavor.

Fill a small, wide-mouthed glass jar with miso. Peel garlic cloves and slice in half lengthwise. Bury each clove in the miso, cover the jar, and refrigerate for one month. At the first signs of a cold, eat one or two cloves daily, rinsing off excess miso first. Use the cloves within two to three months, as garlic does lose its allicin content over time. When you finish the cloves, use the garlic-flavored miso as a delicious soup stock.

Garlic-Lemon Flu Killer

Squeeze three to four fresh lemons, removing the seeds. Slowly bring to a boil. Add one or two cloves of fresh, crushed garlic and reduce heat. Simmer five minutes, stirring occasionally. Add one-eighth to one-quarter cups of honey, one-eighth teaspoon each of nutmeg and cinnamon. Simmer for five more minutes and stir from time to time. Pour into a large mug and serve. It is necessary not only to drink all the liquid, but also to eat the pulp of the lemon and garlic.

Honduran Garlic Cure

Squeeze the juice of one-half lemon into a mug of very hot water. Squash a garlic clove to release its essence and drop it into the lemon water. Add honey to sweeten. Let the mixture steep for a few minutes. Get under the covers, sip slowly, and sweat out your cold.

Latin-American Té

Boil two eucalyptus leaves and one-half stick of cinnamon in one and one-half cups of water for five minutes. Add a tablespoon of honey and the juice of one-half lemon per cup.

Cayenne-Onion Tea

Simmer two teaspoons of chopped fresh cayenne pepper or one-quarter teaspoon cayenne powder and two tablespoons of diced onions in one cup of boiling water for ten minutes. Strain and drink while hot, as needed.

Sinus Cure

For clogged and inflamed sinuses boil one pint of water, add one teaspoon salt, and one teaspoon soda. Cool and add one teaspoon of witch hazel. Sniff up the nose and spit out. Do this several times a day.

Grapefruit Toddy

Squeeze fresh grapefruits to make one and one-half cups. Heat on stove to boiling point. Cool and drink.

Grapefruit Soda Cure

Squeeze the juice from one whole grapefruit. Add honey, if necessary. Pour into large glass. Put one heaping teaspoon of baking soda in another glass. Pour the grapefruit juice into the glass containing baking soda, then *vice-versa*. Pour back and forth, from glass to glass, two or three times over the sink to create a fizzing action. Drink immediately.

Grapefruit Rind Elixir

Cut up a complete grapefruit and place it in a pot containing two cups of water. Boil two or three minutes. Drink warm or cold.

Spicy and Sour Shrimp Soup

At the first signs of a cold, stop at your favorite Thai restaurant and order spicy and sour soup with extra spice. Take it home. Curl up in front of the TV, cover up with a blanket, and eat slowly.

Gypsy Cold Cure

For coughs and colds, combine equal parts of elderberry, crab apple, and blackberry juice. Boil together until a syrup is formed, then add sugar or honey to taste. Take one teaspoonful as needed.

Jewish Princess Cure

Heat one tablespoon olive oil in a stockpot, add one large yellow onion sliced into fine rings, and saute. When the rings begin to separate, add three or four cloves of minced garlic. Add one fifteen-ounce can of chicken stock or broth and one-quarter teaspoon of nutmeg. Bring to a boil, then reduce heat and simmer, covered, for ten minutes. It may not be the genuine article—broth made from a fresh chicken—but princesses like their remedies quick, easy, and delicious.

Marshmallow Leaf Cure

Brew a tea (using the basic tea recipe). Drink up to a quart a day.

Peppermint-Elder Tea

Brew one-half teaspoon each of peppermint and elder leaves (using the basic tea recipe) with one-quarter teaspoon of either yarrow or boneset. This tea also helps to relieve headaches.

Tartar Tea

Dissolve one teaspoon of cream of tartar in one cup of hot water. Drink one cup, two or three times a day, at the first signs of a cold.

Fevergrass/Lemon Grass Tea

The base, stem, and leaves of this grass are used, preferably fresh, for flavoring, especially in the East. Lemon grass (also known as fever grass) is also popular as a "bush herb" among Caribbean people. Similar to citronella and lemon, the leaves make a tea (using basic tea recipe) that alleviates fever and colds. You can also soak in a lemon grass bath (using the basic bath recipe).

Ginger Root Tea

Raw, grated ginger root not only has powerful antibacterial qualities, it heats the body's inner furnace, making it a powerful fighter against cold and flu. The root is a popular remedy used for a variety of ailments in Africa, the Caribbean, and throughout Asia.

Grate one tablespoon of ginger and mix with one cup of water. Heat the mixture *to just before boiling*, then steep for three to five minutes. *Do not allow the ginger water to boil, as this destroys its effectiveness*.

You can brew a big batch of this tea and drink as needed for two days.

Korean Cold Remedy

Put ten slices of fresh ginger root into a large saucepan with four cups of water. Heat almost to boiling, when the ginger turns yellow. Add a cup more of water, two cinnamon sticks, and five or six red dates. (These dates can be found at Asian markets.) Simmer for thirty-five minutes. Store in refrigerator and heat over stove or microwave as needed.

Citrus-Ginger Cold Cure

6 lemons
4 oranges
¼ pound raisins
3 cups honey
3 ounces grated ginger root
1 gallon water

Squeeze the juice from the lemons and oranges and place in the refrigerator. Add all the other ingredients to the water. Bring to a boil and then simmer for an hour. Remove from the heat and pour into a large jar and leave overnight. Add the lemon and orange juice in the morning. Drink two or three cups a day.

Hot Gingered Lemonade

This very delicious and effective blend can be used for almost any autumn or winter imbalances and is especially helpful for colds, influenza, sore throats, congestion, and nausea.

Grate one-quarter cup of fresh ginger root. Add to one quart of water kept just below boiling point, simmer over low heat for five to ten minutes. Remove from heat and add fresh squeezed lemons and honey. (Adjust to taste.) Sprinkle with a pinch of cayenne.

Ginger Root Foot Bath

Another effective use for grated ginger root is as a foot bath. Grate three tablespoons of ginger and place in approximately one quart of water. Heat to just below boiling point, steep for three to five minutes, then cool to the hottest temperature your feet can tolerate. Wrap your body, including your head, in towels or other warm material. Place your feet in the hot ginger water while you sip hot ginger tea, and *sweat*. Go straight to bed. This is an extremely effective cold chaser.

Native American Sage Cure

Pour one cup of boiling water over one teaspoon of sage leaves. Add one teaspoon of cider vinegar, a pinch of cayenne pepper, and honey to taste. Sip cupfuls throughout the day. This is a great fever-buster and also effective relief for night sweats.

Turtle Island Indian Wild Buckwheat Cure

Eat cooked buckwheat throughout the course of the cold. It strengthens your immune system and contains plenty of energy-giving B complex vitamins.

Hot Apple Cider Vinegar and Honey Tea

Vinegar can normalize your digestive juices and combat colds and flus. Combine one cup of hot water with two to three tablespoons of apple cider vinegar and two to three tablespoons of honey. Drink as needed. Do not use if you have a problem with *candida albicans* (yeast infection).

Cold Breaker

Simmer one tablespoon of chopped onion in one cup of barley water (made by simmering one-half cup of barley in one quart of water for twenty minutes) for ten minutes. Remove from heat and add two teaspoons of cod liver oil (or butter or safflower oil). Drink while hot, as needed.

Homemade Nasal Spray

Mix together two cups of water, one teaspoon of salt, and two tablespoons of glycerine. Stir until the salt is completely dissolved. Pour into a sterilized jar with a tightly fitting lid. To use, fill a sterilized atomizer and spray in your nostrils two or three times, as needed.

Herbal Pine Cure

Mix together the following herbs:

> 1 ounce marshmallow root
> ¼ ounce pine needles
> ½ ounce dried mullein flowers

½ ounce sage leaves
½ ounce anise seed

Boil one quart of water and pour it over the herbs. Cover and steep for twenty minutes. Strain and take one-half cup, three times during the day and another before bedtime.

Aloe Juice and Bee Propolis Cure

Gargle with aloe vera juice and take one bee propolis tablet (which has an antiprostaglandin effect, blocking the symptoms of colds and flu). Take three times a day to strike a double blow against sore throats and other cold and flu symptoms. Do not use if you are allergic to bee pollen.

Osha Root

Part of the wild carrot family, osha grows wild in the Rocky Mountains. The root contains the medicinal parts of the plant and should be dug when it is ripe. Chewed or taken in tincture form, it is highly effective relief for sore throats and has beneficial effects on the teeth, digestion, and as an antibacterial agent on skin abrasions and superficial infections. Do not use when pregnant.

Herbal Teas

There are many herbs that make effective cold cures: chamomile, lemon balm, boneset (especially when you have a fever), elder, pennyroyal, and vervain. Use the basic tea recipe.

Rose Hips Delights

The Greeks prepared rose hips (the swelling at the base of the flower that contains the seeds) in many delicious ways. Today, we know rose hips is an effective cold cure because of its high vitamin C content. Brew a tea (using the basic tea recipe). Take as often as needed.

Violets

Roses are red, violets are blue, and while they may not contain as much vitamin C, they are packed with vitamin A, an immune system booster and powerful cold and flu virus opponent. You can brew a tea (using the basic tea recipe), and take as needed. Or you can add the blossoms and chopped leaves to salads and use them as an edible garnish for any dish.

Running Nose Stopper

Steep eight to ten crushed magnolia flowers in one cup of boiled water for ten minutes. Strain and sip as needed.

Goldenseal/Echinacea

Take fifteen to twenty drops of echinacea/goldenseal combination tincture or combine eight to ten drops of each. Take one dose, three times a day. Cut the dose in half for children. You can also buy combination capsules (available at health food stores), one capsule four times a day.

Cold and Flu Tea

Combine one tablespoon each of elder flowers, peppermint, white yarrow, and feverfew. Pour one pint of boiling water over the mixture. Steep for five to ten minutes. Strain, add honey to taste, and drink three to four cups a day.

Ground Ivy Tea

This Gypsy cold and fever remedy is convenient, as it makes use of the ground ivy that grows almost anywhere. Make a tea (using the basic tea recipe), and drink one cup, three times a day.

Alaskan Stuffy Nose Cure

This can only be done when a fresh snow has fallen. Scoop up a handful and plunge your nose into it. Believe it or not, this works—and with no side effects!

If you can't get fresh snow, plunge that clogged-up nose into a basin of cold water.

The cold causes the swollen membranes of your sinuses to contract and expel excess mucus, without the side effects of drugstore cold remedies.

Kitchen Cold Cure

This remedy improves on the Alaskan Stuffy Nose remedy.

Mix together two cups of ice-cold water, one teaspoon of bicarbonate of soda, and one tablespoon of epsom salts. Stir until the soda and salts are completely dissolved. Place a washcloth folded into a square into the solution. Squeeze out excess water and place the cloth over your forehead and the bridge of your nose. Keep dipping the washcloth in the solution to keep it cold until the congestion is relieved.

Reflexologists, who have studied the correspondences between areas of the feet and all the other parts of the body, know that the big toe and the nose correspond. They apply ice water compresses to the big toe or dunk it in ice water in order to relieve congestion in the nose!

Vinegar Steam

This New England folk remedy calls for boiling equal parts of cider vinegar and water in a big pot. Make a hood with a large towel and lean your face over the pot. Inhale the steam to relieve nasal congestion and add germproof moisture.

Clove Steam

Put two teaspoons of cloves in one pint of boiling water. Make a hood with a large towel and lean your face over the pot. Inhale! Make this a double threat against colds and flu by steeping four or five cloves in one cup of boiling water for twenty minutes and drinking that tea after you steam.

Camphor Oil

Dissolve one-half ounce of camphor in two ounces of pure, cold-pressed vegetable oil. Rub around and under the nose.

Camphor-Cayenne Chest Cure

Follow the same recipe as the above, adding one-half teaspoon of cayenne powder. Mix well and rub on your chest.

Spice and Honey Plaster

Mix well the following:

> 2 ounces powdered ginger root
> 1 ounce powdered cinnamon
> ½ ounce powdered mustard
> 2 teaspoons red pepper

Add enough honey to make a smooth consistency. Spread on a soft cloth and apply to your chest. Secure and leave on overnight.

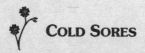

Cold Sores

Cold sores are caused by an internal viral infection called herpes simplex I, which resides permanently in the body. Cold sores generally appear when your body's immune powers are low and the virus activates. But you can speed the healing of cold sores by dabbing on a few drops of any of the following tinctures: calendula, goldenseal, hypericum, and myrrh.

Sage Tea

Brewed according to the basic tea recipe, sage will help shorten the outbreak. Drink one cup, three times a day.

Tea Tree Oil

Dab one drop of tea tree oil on the cold sore, twice daily, morning and night. Essential oil of lavender can also be dabbed onto the sore.

COLIC

Anise or Fennel Tea

One to two ounces of either of these sweet-tasting teas (using the basic tea recipe) can be given to your baby in a bottle or dropper.

Chamomile Tea

Brewed according to the basic tea recipe, this especially mild yet powerfully effective herbal drink soothes and calms baby's delicate intestines.

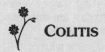

COLITIS

If you suspect you suffer from this chronic inflammatory condition of the lower bowel, see your doctor before using any of the following remedies.

Slippery Elm Implant

Mix one ounce of slippery elm powder with one pint of boiling water. Steep for twenty to thirty minutes. Cool and strain. Inject into the bowel with a rectal syringe or enema device. Many natural healers claim this works where all others have failed.

Amish Slippery Elm Milk

Mix one teaspoon of slippery elm powder into a glass of hot milk. Drink or use with cereal. Do not use if you are lactose intolerant, a common condition in those suffering from colitis.

Marshmallow Combination Tea

Combine the following:

> 1 ounce marshmallow root
> ½ ounce lady's slipper or valerian root
> ¼ ounce slippery elm

Mix well and boil in two pints of water for fifteen minutes. Strain while warm. Take one-half cup every two hours throughout the day. Do not expect instant results; this remedy works over the long term.

Fenugreek Tea

This tea soothes the irritated bowel linings of those suffering from colitis and helps the body to expel gas and excess mucus.

Pour one cup of boiling water over two teaspoons of fenugreek tea. Steep for five to ten minutes. Strain and drink one cup, three to four times a day.

Banana Milk

Mash a banana and mix the pulp and the skin with one pint of milk. Boil for twenty minutes. Cool and drink as needed. Do not use this remedy if you are lactose intolerant.

Pears

Eat pears freely to relieve colitis.

Saint John's Wort Tea

This works well on mild cases of colitis. Pour one cup of boiling water over one teaspoon of dried herb. Strain. Take one cup, three times a day.

Goldenseal Suppositories

Mix together one ounce each of goldenseal powder, boric acid, and white flour. Add enough glycerin to be able to shape the mixture into suppositories. Insert at bedtime. The suppository will be eliminated along with your morning bowel movement.

Psyllium Seeds

Soak one teaspoon of the seeds overnight in water, and take in the morning with breakfast. Or take one teaspoon of powdered psyllium seeds with one cup of juice.

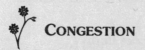

CONGESTION

Peach Leaf Syrup

Simmer one leaf per one cup of boiling water. Cool, strain, and add enough honey to make a syrup. Take one tablespoon, as needed, to clear congestion and soothe irritated membranes.

Nettle Leaf Tea

Brew a tea of nettle leaves (using the basic tea recipe). Take one cup, three or four times a day, to rid the stomach, urinary tract, and lungs of excess mucus.

Eucalyptus Steam

Boil a large pot of water. Remove from heat and add a few drops of eucalyptus oil. Make a tent with a towel and lean over the pot, breathing in the vapors until they dissipate.

Ice Socks

Wring out a pair of cotton socks in ice water before you retire for the evening. Put them on and cover them with heavy wool socks. Leave on overnight.

Olive Oil–Garlic Poultice

Rub the bottoms of your feet with olive oil. Mash up enough garlic to make a poultice one-quarter inch thick that will cover both soles. Place between layers of gauze and tape to feet. Cover with socks and leave on overnight.

Mustard Seed Foot Bath

Steep one tablespoon of ground mustard seeds per quart of boiling water. When the temperature cools sufficiently, place your feet in the solution to draw the blood away from your congested nose and chest to the lower parts of the body.

Mustard Plaster

Mix one part ground mustard seeds with four parts whole wheat flour. Add enough egg white to turn it into a thick paste. Apply to chest, cover, and secure well.

Fenugreek Tea

These seeds dissolve mucus, making them a valuable decongestive aid for the entire body, whether the cause of congestion is a cold or flu virus, pollution, or an allergic reaction. You can chew the seeds or brew a tea to drink and to use as a gargle. In some cultures, those with mucus-clogged sinuses inhale the tea, then throw their heads back to allow the tea to circulate through their sinus cavities.

Add two teaspoons of fenugreek seeds to one cup of boiling water. Steep for five minutes, then stir well, and strain. Add honey and/or lemon juice to taste.

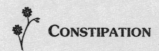 **CONSTIPATION**

Chronic constipation usually indicates an underlying condition that should be diagnosed before treating. If constipation is chronic, consult your doctor. It could be indicative of anything from an allergy to a disease of the colon to a lack of sufficient fiber in your diet.

Mulberry Leaf Tea

Brew a tea from the dried or fresh mulberry leaves (using the basic tea recipe). Drink one cup, three times a day, or as needed. (Mulberry *root* tea is used to cure diarrhea.)

Aloe Vera Juice

Drink a glass of aloe vera juice three times a day. It can be purchased at your local health food store with natural sweetening flavors added.

Agar-Agar

This mineral-rich gelatin comes from seaweed and its mucilaginous quality makes it excellent as a laxative. Agar-agar is

used by those who follow a macrobiotic diet to make puddings, gelatins, or simply as a thickener for other dishes.

Mix the agar-agar with water and drink—one teaspoon per
one cup of water. Use it as a thickener when making your
desserts.

Laxative Fruits

Certain fruits are also effective in improving elimination. Apples, pears, persimmons, pineapples, stewed rhubarb, and
dried prunes are all beneficial.

Intestinal Cleanser

Combine the following:

> 1 cup aloe vera juice
> 4 tablespoons blackberry concentrate
> ⅓ cup flaxseed
> 1 teaspoon slippery elm powder
> ½ cup agar-agar flakes
> 1 cup water

Place all the ingredients in a pot and bring to a boil. Lower
the heat and simmer until the mixture reaches a thick, gravy-
like consistency. Allow it cool, then place it in a container
and chill until the mixture is firm. Cut into one inch squares.
Take two squares daily on an empty stomach until normal
bowel function is restored.

Agar-Agar and Flaxseed Jelly

Add one teaspoon of agar-agar and one teaspoon of flaxseed
to one pint of boiling water. Simmer for five minutes. Cool.
The mixture will jell. Take one or two teaspoons of the jelly
before meals. You can also use fruit juice in place of the
water.

Tamarind Jam

Mix together the following:

> ½ ounce tamarind pulp
> 1 ounce honey
> 1 ounce raspberries or strawberries

Take two teaspoons twice a day, in the morning and the evening.

Fig Tea

Boil together two ounces each of figs, raisins, and barley in two pints of water for fifteen minutes. Add one-half ounce of powdered licorice root, letting it soak into the mixture for a few minutes. Cool, stir, then strain. Take one-half cup, two times a day, morning and evening.

Fenugreek Milk

Brew the roots, stalks, and seeds of fenugreek into a strong decoction (using the basic decoction recipe). Add one-half cup to one cup of boiled milk. Drink when cool for a laxative that also heals irritated bowel linings.

Fruit Combination Laxative

Chop coarsely one-half ounce each of cooked prunes and cooked figs. Add one cup of blackstrap molasses. Steep one ounce of senna leaves in one pint of boiling water for twenty minutes. Strain and add the liquid to the fruit-molasses mixture. Simmer until the figs and prunes become a pulp. Take one or two tablespoons before bedtime. Children can take two teaspoons.

Gooseberry-Fig Mash

Mix together equal parts of figs and gooseberries. Mash well or blend at low speed in the blender. Take one tablespoon twice a day, morning and evening, for a gentle laxative that also expels worms.

Fig Paste

Figs have a laxative effect because of the bulk of the seeds and fiber, as well as a solvent in the juice. Eat dried or fresh figs freely or make fig paste.
  Combine the following:

> 3 ounces figs
> 3 ounces raisins
> ⅓ ounce powdered senna pods
> 1 ounce ground linseed

  Mix ingredients together and pulverize. Shape the resulting paste into small rolls and store in the refrigerator. Eat the rolls as needed.

Blackstrap Molasses

This old American remedy for constipation is still a good one, and it provides you with minerals and B vitamins. Take one or two tablespoons before bedtime. If you wish, you can stir the molasses into a glass of milk, juice, or water.
  Honey is a milder remedy for constipation. You might want to use half honey, half blackstrap molasses.

Yogurt-Fruit Treat

Combine one cup of plain yogurt, five well-chopped prunes, and two tablespoons of blackstrap molasses. Mix thoroughly in a blender and take before bed or as a part of your breakfast meal.

Mild Laxative Tea

In cases of chronic constipation, dandelion, taken as a tea or in capsule or tincture forms, acts as a mild, non–habit-forming laxative while it promotes healthy circulation and restores gastric balance. Licorice tea or tincture is also effective in mild cases.

Gypsy Nettle Cure

Boil one tablespoon of nettles in one pint of milk for fifteen minutes. Drink one cup at bedtime, or more if needed.

Seed Laxative

Combine equal parts of psyllium seed, flax seed, and chia seed. Soak two to three tablespoons overnight in one cup of tea made from equal parts raisins and licorice. Take three tablespoons in the morning. Repeat every hour, until the condition is relieved.

Bowel Regulating Pellets

This tea remedies both conditions of constipation and diarrhea.
    Combine the following herb powders:

> 6 teaspoons rhubarb root
> 1 teaspoon slippery elm
> 1 teaspoon cinnamon

Add enough water to make a paste. Form pea-sized pills. Dry in an oven with low heat, then dip in melted beeswax. Take two to six pills, three times a day.

Olive Oil

One tablespoon or more of olive oil acts as a mild, natural laxative that also soothes irritated bowel linings. Take alone or mix it into your salad dressing.

Nettles

Though nettles are used to stop diarrhea, they are also helpful for constipation. Pick young spring nettles and boil a handful in one pint of milk. Drink cupfuls as needed.

 # CORNS

A good way to prepare for any of the following treatments is to soak your feet first in a small plastic tub of hot water and one-half cup of epsom salts or baking soda.

Sure-Fire Corn Remover

Chop an onion finely and place it in a plastic bag. Pull the bag over the toe and secure it well, but not too tightly, with tape or a rubber band. Leave it on overnight.

Dandelion Corn and Wart Cure

Squeeze the broken stem of a leaf or flower until the milky juice extrudes. Apply to the corn (or wart) and let it dry. Repeat this for three days in a row until the corn (or wart) falls off.

Castor Oil

Apply castor oil often to calluses and corns to soften them and relieve the pain. Frequent applications will also prevent the formation of corns and calluses.

A variation calls for mixing baking soda and castor oil, then applying in the same manner.

Beer Yeast Poultice

Spread the yeast from beer on a clean cloth or gauze. Apply to corn and tape securely. Do this every day, for three or four weeks, and the corn will disappear.

If you can't get beer yeast, use brewer's yeast moistened with lemon juice. Spread it on cotton or cloth and bind securely.

Black Bread Poultice

Soak a piece of Russian black bread in vinegar, then bind it to the corn.

American Indian Ivy Leaf Poultice

Bruise ivy leaves and soak overnight in vinegar. Place on a clean cloth or gauze and apply to corn. Leave on all day or all night. Repeat until the pain goes away and the corn softens.

Lemon Remover

Soak your feet in hot water just before bedtime. Dry them thoroughly. Take a small piece of lemon peel with the pulp intact and bind it over the corn or callus. Some people prefer to use a slice of lemon. Bandage it and leave it on overnight. Remove in the morning. Repeat for four or five days, after which you can peel off the growth. (Orange rind can also be used.)

Yarrow Foot Bath

Add one cup of yarrow leaves and one tablespoon of salt to three quarts of hot water. Soak for at least twenty to thirty minutes. This will soften any corn, callus, or bunion, and allow it to slough off.

Castor Oil Rub

Rub castor oil on calluses frequently to soften them. Olive oil can also be used. It is also effective for dry skin, corns that are just forming, and for dry and/or splitting nails.

Hawaiian Corn Cure

Slice a *fresh* pineapple thinly or grate it. Place the pineapple in a clean cloth or gauze and apply over the corn. Tape well and leave it on overnight. Repeat until relief is obtained.

Papaya Juice

This healing juice, either applied directly or with a clean cloth or piece of gauze, dissolves corns and warts.

Vinegar Soak

Soak a piece of gauze or a small piece of cloth in cider vinegar. Bind to the corn and leave on for twenty-four hours. The corn should fall off, including the root.

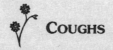

COUGHS

Do not suppress a cough unless it brings nothing up. If you are coughing and bringing up phlegm, let it out! The purpose of coughing is to keep the lungs and breathing passages free from dust, infective agents, and mucus, eliminating whatever is impeding healing. Herbs can be used to reduce the discomfort of a cough and aid in the healing process in three ways: Most respiratory herbs are *demulcents* which contain *mucilage*, a slimy substance that resembles mucus. This "mucus" helps soothe inflamed tissues and aids the natural mucus in its work. *Expectorants* promote the secretion of natural mucus. They help to moisten inflamed tissue and also water down thick mucus, making a cough more effective. *Respiratory sedatives* suppress the cough reflex. Use them only when coughing is interfering with sleep or is exhausting. Antiviral and antibacterial herbs are also useful in remedies for coughs that accompany infections. Many cough remedies use honey, which should not be given to children under one year of age.

Classic Cough Syrup

Combine the following:

> ½ cup fenugreek seeds
> ½ cup raisins
> 10 dried figs
> 5 cups water

Bring to a boil, then lower the flame and simmer for thirty to forty minutes. Cool and strain. Store in the refrigerator and take as much as you want, as often as needed.

Mullein Cough Syrup

Simmer one cup of crushed mullein leaves in one quart of boiling water until the liquid becomes a thick syrup. Add honey to taste. Take one tablespoon every hour, or as needed, until symptoms abate.

Horehound-Licorice Cough Syrup

Combine one quart of horehound with one quart of water and boil down to one pint. Add three sticks of licorice and a few drops of lemon essence. Take one tablespoon, three times a day.

Horseradish-Horehound Syrup

Simmer one ounce of grated horseradish root and three ounces of horehound in three cups of water until the liquid is reduced by half. Strain and add one-half cup of honey. Take one or two teaspoons as needed.

Gypsy Cough Cure

For colds, coughs, and bronchitis, Gypsies eat chopped horseradish. You can add it to vegetable juices or eat it as a condiment on virtually any food.

Garlic-Horseradish Cough Remedy

Mix together one-half cup honey, one tablespoon minced garlic, and one teaspoon of fresh, grated horseradish. Take one or two teaspoons as needed.

Fig Cough Syrup

Drop two ounces of fig tree leaves in two pints of boiling water. Continue at a low boil for twenty minutes. Add one-half cup of honey. Strain when cool. Take one tablespoonful as needed.

Fig-Barley Water

Prepare barley water by boiling one cup of barley in one quart of pure water for twenty to thirty minutes. Strain out the barley. Using the barley water, boil one-half cup of figs for twenty to thirty minutes. Strain. Use the water for any pulmonary complaint.

Sage, Garlic, and Honey Tea

Boil six cups of water and pour over the following: two heaping tablespoons of sage leaves, two cloves of finely chopped organic garlic, and one-half lemon. Steep for five minutes. Drink as much as you can while bundled in bed, and you will sweat out any upper respiratory infection.

Thyme Steam

This is a wonderful ritual for chest colds, or when you wake up feeling congested. One of my favorite blends contains the following:

> 2 tablespoons thyme
> 1 tablespoon sage
> 1 tablespoon rosemary
> 1 tablespoon lavender

Pour boiling water into a large bowl over a handful of the fresh or dried herbal blend. Lean your head over the bowl and make a tent from a towel. Inhale slowly, relax, and let the steam do its work. (Makes a great facial, too!)

Thyme Tea

Thyme (thymol extract) is the main ingredient in Listerine because it's an effective respiratory antiseptic when you are coughing up yellow mucus. Steep one teaspoon of thyme in one cup of boiling water. This tea is also an old remedy for headaches.

Thyme-Honey Cough Syrup

Make a strong thyme tea by placing three tablespoons of dried thyme leaves (not powdered thyme) into a quart glass jar. Add one pint of boiling water and close the lid. Let steep until cool. Strain and add one cup of honey. Stir well. Refrigerate this mixture and it will keep for several months. Take one teaspoon every hour to relieve a cough.

Obstinate Cough Chaser

Place one tablespoon of whole flaxseed in a quart of boiling water. Simmer for one-half hour, then bring to boil again and pour over two ounces of fresh or dried thyme and three to four lemon slices. Sweeten with honey or barley sugar. Strain when cold, and take one tablespoon of the mixture, five or six times a day.

Baked Onion

Onions are antiinflammatory and honey is a natural expectorant, promoting the free flow of mucus.

Peel one whole onion and squeeze out the juice. Mix the juice with honey and swallow as hot as possible. Or you can simply slice an onion and eat it raw. Or inhale its fumes which are said to benefit bronchitis, asthma, and other respiratory ailments. You can also crush onions, mix them with a camphorated oil, and spread them over a warm flannel. Apply to the chest and back. Or you can slice the onions, fry them until they're brown, cool to a tolerable temperature, and place them between two washcloths or pieces of clean cloth and use as a chest poultice.

Onion-Honey-Pine Cough Syrup

This remedy relieves coughs and kills the germs. Mix together one cup each of honey and water. Add one-half cup of chopped onions and one-third cup of pine tree buds. Bring to a boil, then cover and simmer for twenty minutes. Take one tablespoon as needed; children take one- to two-teaspoon doses.

Southern Honeysuckle Comfort Tea

Make a strong tea (using two teaspoons to one cup of water) from honeysuckle leaves and flowers. This tea soothes irritated mucus membranes and helps expel phlegm.

Dry Cough Tea

This tea combines the expectorant and demulcent qualities of mullein, the antiinflammatory and adrenal toning quality of licorice, and the carminative, antispasmodic, and nervine properties of peppermint. Very effective!

> 1 tablespoon of mullein
> ½ tablespoon licorice
> ½ tablespoon peppermint

Mix well and brew a tea (using the basic tea recipe). Steep for ten to fifteen minutes. Drink slowly. Take one cup, three or four times a day.

Marshmallow Tea

This tea is effective for dry or inflamed coughs high in the respiratory tract accompanied by a sore throat. Combined with honey, the dry root of this demulcent herb contains up to one-third mucilage by weight. Marshmallow is also an expectorant, so the double action of the plant mucilage and the increased natural mucus will help soothe inflamed membranes.

Cover one ounce of chopped marshmallow root with one pint of cold water and let it sit overnight. Add two tablespoons of honey to one cup of the marshmallow water. Sip as often as desired throughout the day.

Black Currant Cough Syrup

Simmer two heaping teaspoons of black currants in two cups of boiling water for ten minutes. Strain and add honey to taste. Take by the tablespoon, as needed.

Red Cherry Stew

Cover ripe, red cherries in enough water to stew over a low heat. Add honey to taste. Remove the pits when cool and add lemon juice for a nice tartness. Take by the tablespoon, as desired.

Plum Tea

Plums, known for their laxative effect, are also effective remedies against bronchitis. Brew the tea, using a handful of plums to one quart of water. Simmer for twenty minutes. Strain off the plums (and eat them separately), and drink the remaining plum tea freely.

Lemon Syrup

Mix together the following:

> 1 thinly sliced lemon
> ½ pint flaxseeds
> 2 ounces honey

Simmer the mixture in one quart of water for four hours. Cool and strain. Pour into one pint bottle and add water if the mixture doesn't fill the bottle. Take one tablespoon, four times a day, and more if coughing is severe.

Honey-Turnip Syrup

Scrub, but do not peel, a large white turnip. Slice off the bottom so that it is flat and even. Cut in half and divide each half into three or four slices. Cover each slice with honey and then assemble the slices in a stack so that they form a whole turnip standing on one end. Let stand overnight. In the morning, the turnip juice and honey will have formed a syrup that stops a cough in its tracks.

American Indian Mullein-Molasses Cough Syrup

Simmer a handful of mullein leaves in one pint of liquid made of equal parts water and molasses. Cook at low heat until a syrup results. Take by the tablespoon as needed.

American Indian Bark Tea

Make a tea (using the basic decoction recipe) from the inner bark of white pine. Take by the cupful as needed. The bark of wild cherry tree can also be used.

Slippery Elm Tea

Slippery elm is great medicine, with a soothing and strengthening effect on both the digestive and respiratory tracts. The unsweetened tea (using the basic tea recipe) is effective for all pulmonary complaints, including coughs and bronchitis. And if you are also suffering from gastric complaints, it will work on them as well!

Red Clover Tea

This old American Indian remedy, made from the red clover blossoms (using the basic tea recipe) helps asthma, hoarseness, colds, coughs, and general respiratory irritation. Add honey and a squeeze of lemon. Sip hot, every hour or two.

Red Clover Cough Syrup

The Indians also liked to make a strong syrup of red clover, mixing the blossoms with equal parts of the juice of roasted onions and honey. Heat one pint of honey with one pint of water to boiling. Add one ounce of red clover blossoms and the juice of one roasted onion. Simmer for fifteen minutes. Let stand until cool, then refrigerate and use as needed. The resulting mixture is effective for colds, coughs, hoarseness, and any irritation of the lungs, windpipe, and bronchial tubes. You can also make the syrup without onion.

Pureed Rose Hips

Place two pounds of clean rose hips into one and one-half pints of boiling water. Cover and bring to boil again. Simmer for fifteen to twenty minutes. Blend at a low speed in a blender. Take one to two tablespoons as needed, especially at bedtime, to soothe your throat and prevent coughing.

Rose Hips Dessert Syrup

To make this delicious syrup, use pureed rose hips, fruit juice, and honey. Mix together the following:

> ½ cup pureed rose hips
> ½ cup orange or pineapple juice
> 3 tablespoons honey
> 2 teaspoons lemon juice

Bring the puree, fruit juice, and honey to a boil. Add lemon juice. Use as a topping and take one or two tablespoons as needed to soothe your throat and prevent coughing.

Violet Syrup

Mix together the following:

> ½ pound fresh or dried violets and stems
> 2 cups water
> 1 cup honey
> ¼ cup almond oil

Bring the water to a boil. Place the violets in a jar into which you pour the boiling water. Cover and let steep overnight. Strain out the violets, add honey, and return to the stove. Allow the mixture to come almost, but not quite, to a boil. Add the almond oil and mix well. Cool and pour into a jar or bottle. Cap tightly. Take one or two tablespoons to soothe your throat and prevent coughing.

Mango Juice

This fruit is awkward to juice. If you can't get it fresh, buy it by the bottle in your health food store. Drink freely to help cure all kinds of respiratory disorders.

Lemon-Linseed Remedy

Simmer two tablespoons of whole linseeds in one quart of water for one hour and fifteen minutes. Strain. Add the juice from two lemons and one-half cup of honey. Take by the tablespoon, as needed.

Peach Leaf Tea

Steep one teaspoon of crushed green peach tree leaves in two quarts of boiling water for at least ten minutes. Cool and strain. Take one tablespoon with a few drops of honey every hour, until symptoms abate.

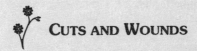

CUTS AND WOUNDS

Minor cuts and wounds should be treated with natural antiseptics to avoid infection. Make sure the injured area is cleaned of any sand, dirt, or splinters before using substances that close up the area. To speed up healing, expose smaller cuts to the fresh air as often as possible.

Plantain Poultice

Macerate the roots and leaves and add water to form a paste. Apply to wounds, cuts, or inflammations, and cover.

Comfrey Root Poultice

Mix ground comfrey root with enough water to make a poultice that promotes healing and helps close wounds.

Green Dressing

This dressing heals wounds and acts as an antibiotic to prevent and cure infection. Combine pulped comfrey leaves with enough honey to make a spreadable paste. Add one small minced garlic clove per each tablespoon of the comfrey-honey mixture for germ-killing action. Mix well and spread on a piece of gauze cut to cover the wound. Place over affected area and bind securely. Replace the dressing as the drawing, healing, and antiseptic qualities draw out impurities and inflammation.

Papaya Juice

Apply the juice directly to the cut or soak a clean cloth or piece of gauze and cover the affected area. This juice will promote healing at the same time it destroys scars without harming healthy tissue.

Papaya Leaves

The Seminole Indians would wrap ulcerated skin and wounds with papaya leaves to promote healing without scar tissue.

Pepper

As odd as it sounds, cayenne pepper stops bleeding and does not burn. Put a little of the ground pepper in a wound. Honey also stops bleeding and has antiseptic properties.

Essential Oil Antibiotic

Combine the following essential oils:

> 2 drops tea tree
> 5 drops lavender
> 2 cups water

Bathe the area with this solution, then place two drops of lavender oil on a gauze bandage and cover the cut. Do this twice daily.

Daisy Poultice

Place one pint of daisy leaves in the blender with enough witch hazel to make a pulp. Spread on cuts, wounds, bruises (and most other skin disorders). Cover with gauze or clean cloth and tape well.

Honeysuckle Lotion

This remedy was a favorite of the American Indians for healing all types of wounds and sores. Cook fresh honeysuckle leaves in water (using the basic tea recipe) over a low heat for at least twenty minutes. Strain and apply to affected area.

For more severe wounds, pulp the honeysuckle leaves and apply to affected area. Cover with gauze or clean cloth and tape securely.

Fenugreek Seed Compress

This compress is effective in treating deep gashlike wounds in danger of infection. Moisten the seeds slightly, then grind them into a thick paste, either with the blender or a mortar and pestle. Spread a thick layer on a clean piece of cloth or gauze and attach securely to the wound. Leave on, changing the dressing, as it draws out infection.

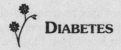 **DIABETES**

Blood sugar problems are alleviated by a strict high protein, low carbohydrate diet of four to six meals daily. Include regular servings of oatmeal, dried beans, kelp, and artichokes. The following remedies also help to stabilize the blood sugar problems that lead to diabetes.

Red Clover and Dandelion Tea

Mix together equal parts of red clover blossoms and powdered dandelion root. Pour one cup of boiling water over one teaspoon of the herb mixture. Steep for at least ten minutes. Drink at least one cup, three times a day.

Blueberry and Huckleberry Leaf Tea

Huckleberry and blueberry leaf teas are old American Indian remedies for diabetes that are still being studied today. Research shows that the leaves of these berries contain myrtilin, a substance that dissolves blood sugar. The berries themselves are mineral-rich and purify the blood. They also tone and strengthen the pancreas.

Steep one teaspoon of dried, cut blueberry or huckleberry leaves in one cup of hot water. Take every six hours to help stablize blood sugar.

Peach or Strawberry Leaf Tea

Brew a basic tea, using one peach or strawberry leaf per one cup of boiling water for benefits similar to the above teas. Drink one cup, three times a day.

Pau D'Arco Tea

Boil one teaspoon of this bark in one cup of water for ten minutes, then steep for ten minutes more. Drink one cup, three times a day, to lower your blood sugar.

Avocado/Eucalyptus/Walnut Tea

Pour one cup of boiling water over one-quarter avocado leaf, one eucalyptus leaf, and one walnut tree leaf. Steep for at least ten minutes. Drink one cup, three times a day.

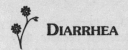

DIARRHEA

Chronic diarrhea suggests an underlying condition that should be diagnosed before treating. If diarrhea is persistent, consult your doctor. It could be indicative of anything from an allergy to food poisoning, viral, parasitic, or bacterial infection, or a disease of the colon.

Cinnamon Cayenne Tea

Bring two cups of water to a boil. Add one-quarter teaspoon of cinnamon (one-eighth for small children) and a dash of cayenne pepper. Simmer for twenty minutes. Cool, strain, and sip as needed.

Barley Water

Boil one cup of barley to one quart of water until the barley is tender. Strain. Use the barley as a food and drink the water to check diarrhea. Take one cup as needed.

Welsh Hot Poker in Milk Cure

This interesting folk remedy is patterned after a homeopathic remedy, iron, which is prescribed for diarrhea. Or did the homeopathic remedy come from this folk cure? Place an iron poker in a burning fireplace until it is red-hot. Then dip it in a cup of milk for about thirty seconds. Sip the milk slowly. The iron in the poker charges the milk with healing properties. In any case, boiled milk is another remedy for diarrhea. That is, unless you are lactose-intolerant.

Bananas

Bananas are helpful, not only because they are rich in pectin, a binding substance, but because they contain potassium, magnesium, and other nutrients that are lost in diarrhea.

Banana Milk

Mash a banana and mix the pulp and the skin with one pint of milk. Boil for twenty minutes. Cool and drink as needed.

Bayberry

Taken in capsule or tea form (made according to the standard recipe), bayberry combats the debilitating effects of diarrhea. It has a soothing effect and acts as an astringent to clean and tone the bowels. Blackberries, eaten by the handful, are also helpful, as are teas made from huckleberry leaves, slippery elm, red raspberry leaf, myrrh, white oat bark, and peppermint.

Catnip Tea

Taken in capsule or tea form (using the basic tea recipe), this is an excellent antispasmodic to stop cramps and gripping pain.

Blackberry Root Tea

Use for more severe cases. Boil two tablespoons of dried powdered roots in one and one-half pints of water for twenty minutes, or until the mixture boils down to one pint. Take one-half cup every two hours, until the diarrhea stops. Other soothing, nourishing teas that will also tighten the bowels include ginger root (freshly grated is best, simmered for twenty minutes), mullein, nettle (simmer for ten minutes), and elder flowers (brew for five minutes).

Blackberry Cordial

Mix together the following:

>1 cup ripe blackberries
>2 cups raw sugar
>3 cloves
>2 small sticks of cinnamon
>1 pint hot water

Boil together for ten minutes. Cool, then strain. Add port wine in an amount equal to the liquid. Take one tablespoon in one-half cup of warm water, as needed.

Apple Cure

To stop an attack of diarrhea in its tracks, peel, core, and shred an apple. Let the apple turn brown—this takes about twenty minutes—then eat. Do this every two hours, taking no other food, until the diarrhea stops. The apple must be brown to have the desired effect.

Arrow Root

A popular root used in a powder form by country folk for centuries, it yields a pure, nutritive form of starch, helpful in diarrhea. High in carbohydrates, arrow root also makes a good drink for convalescents.

Vanilla Rice Cure

Boil one quart of water and add one-third cup of rice. Simmer for twenty minutes, then add three drops of vanilla extract and honey to taste. Sprinkle with cinnamon powder. Strain and drink the liquid.

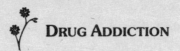

DRUG ADDICTION

Drug addiction drains the body of mineral salts, depletes its store of vitamins, and disturbs hormone balance and function. Symptoms of withdrawal usually include convulsive shaking, quivering, nausea, vomiting, and diarrhea, as the body attempts to rid itself of accumulated toxins. For this reason, natural healers recommend that these symptoms not be overly suppressed by other drugs. Enemas are recommended to speed up the cleansing process.

The following remedies support the body's attempt to rid itself of poisons. But any of the following recommendations should be used in tandem with your doctor's recommendations.

Milk Thistle Seeds

Taken in extract or capsule form, this seed can help repair damage to a liver that has been overexposed to chemicals, drugs, or alcohol. Take according to bottle instructions.

Chamomile-Hops Tea

Brew equal parts of hops and chamomile (using the basic tea recipe) to treat alcoholics suffering from delirium tremens and drug addicts with nervous exhaustion. Drink as needed to soothe and calm.

Blessed Thistle

Taken in capsule form—one, three times a day—this detoxing herb is effective for anyone detoxing from drugs or hepatitis or mononucleosis. (It is also very nourishing for the female organs and women who are breast-feeding.)

Hops Tea

Brew hops tea (using the basic tea recipe) and add one-quarter teaspoon of cayenne pepper. Drink three to four cups a day to help reduce the craving for alcohol and settle queasy stomachs.

Withdrawal Tea

This tea helps soothes nerves when withdrawing from drugs or alcohol. Combine equal parts of lady's slipper and skullcap. Make a tea (using the basic tea recipe). Take one-quarter cup, every hour. As symptoms lessen, take the tea less and less frequently.

Russian-American Cures for Drug Addiction

L.S.D.

Mix a tablespoon of each of powdered gotu kola and slippery elm with enough honey and a little milk to make a paste. For one week, take this mixture two to three times a day, alternating with natural diuretics such as parsley tea or the combination tea recipe given below. Skip treatment the second week, then resume every third day for the third week.

Natural Diuretic Tea: Mix together equal parts of dandelion, birchleaf, buchu, and uva ursi. Using the basic tea recipe, steep for ten minutes in boiling water. Drink three to four cups a day. During this time, drink chamomile tea to soothe nerves. If highly agitated, drink linden tea.

Heroin

Heroin does not produce severe constipation, so a daily dose of slippery elm is enough to keep the bowels moving and soothe irritated mucus linings. Add a dash of cayenne pepper to food every day to stimulate body functions. Drink any mint tea with the juice of one-half lemon and honey as often as possible, along with a diuretic tea such as uva ursi or bilberry leaf. Irish moss helps with the respiratory problems heroin often causes.

Marijuana

Drink one cup each of chamomile tea and wood betony (using the basic tea recipe) to soothe nerves. Do not use caffeinated tea, coffee, or white sugar. Use sea salt only, eat meat at least two times a week, and eat a dish of lentils and onions at least once a day. Chew one clove of garlic each day, or one-half raw onion and one raw leek. Eat green salad three times a day. Take psyllium pods (senna) every third day for nine days. Drink one cup of tea made from equal parts sarsaparilla tea and blessed thistle (doubling the amount of herb used in the basic recipe) twice a day, every other day for one month, to cleanse and prevent depression.

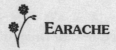

EARACHE

Oatmeal Earache Cure

Heat oatmeal, sand, or salt in a pan. Pour the oatmeal into a sock and knot it. Heat in microwave for thirty to forty-five seconds. (Make sure it's not too hot and the heat is distributed uniformly.) Place the sock over the infected ear. It conforms to the shape of the ear far better than a heating pad.

Potato Earache Cure

Bake one large baking potato for forty minutes. Wrap in a thin towel and hold over ear. The potato does not conform to the ear, but it holds heat for a long time. You can also bake an onion until soft, wrap it in a layer of cheesecloth, and hold it against the affected ear.

Garlic Earache Cure

To ''unplug'' ears and combat infection, mix one drop of olive or safflower oil with a pinch of grated garlic. Wrap securely inside a tiny square of cheesecloth and place inside ear. Leave in overnight. Some remedies call for stewing the garlic in the oil, straining, and then placing a few drops in your ear every day, followed with a plug of cotton. It is helpful to also drink pleurisy root tea.

Peach Leaf Cure

Steep a peach leaf (using one leaf per one cup of boiling water) for ten minutes. Cool, strain well, and place a few drops, using a medicinal dropper, into the infected ear.

Lobelia Earache Cure

Two drops of lobelia tincture in each ear relieves the pain almost immediately.

Tea Tree Cure

Place one drop of tea tree oil on a small ball of cotton and place in the ear overnight.

Oil of Roses Gypsy Cure

Mix three drops each of oil of roses and apple cider vinegar. Place in the affected ear. Make a bag from gauze into which you place equal parts of chamomile and melilot oil. Place the bag *over* your ear.

Hot/Cold Cure

This treatment sounds extreme, but it relieves pain and promotes circulation to the affected area. Place a washcloth in ice water. Place another washcloth in very hot water. Wring out the hot washcloth and hold to the ear for three minutes. Wring out the cold washcloth and hold to the ear for thirty seconds. Repeat until symptoms subside.

Plantain Leaf Extract

This remedy is supposed to heal almost all ear complaints and sharpen hearing. Make or purchase plantain extract (using the basic tincture recipe). Take twenty to thirty drops in one-half cup of water, three to four times a day.

Chamomile Oil Drops

To prepare the oil, place three ounces of chamomile flowers in one and one-half pints of pure vegetable oil. Simmer in a glass or stainless steel saucepan for forty minutes. Remove from heat and let stand overnight. Strain and bottle. Place a few warm drops in irritated, infected ears.

Molasses Pain Reliever

Dip a small cotton ball in blackstrap molasses and stuff into your ears overnight.

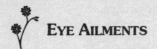 **EYE AILMENTS**

Swollen Eye Reducer

Grate a white potato. You can place it directly on your eyes, but it's less messy if you put it between two clean pieces of cheesecloth and cover the eye. Leave on for at least fifteen minutes.

Sty Eliminator

This one comes from a Brooklyn-born friend of my parents. It may seem strange but this method has always worked for me, if I use it as soon as I feel a sty coming on. Spit on your clean finger and dab the spit in your eye. Repeat until you no longer feel the sty.

Eye Strain and Sty Compress

Make a tea (using the basic tea recipe) of chamomile flowers. Strain and chill. Soak two cotton pads in the tea and place over your eyes for twenty minutes. You can do the same with two chamomile tea bags by dipping them in boiling water, then putting them in the freezer to chill and applying to your eyes. However, herbs bought in tea bag form tend to have lost much of their medicinal properties.

Green Tea Soother

Simply moisten the tea bags in boiling water and use as compresses. This is also effective for stys that have come to a head to ease the irritation and help them empty.

Burdock Sty Chaser

Prepare a strong decoction (doubling the amount of burdock root in the basic decoction recipe). Take one tablespoon, three to four times a day.

Irish-American Cabbage Sty Chaser

In the heyday of Hollywood glamour, movie queens used this remedy to clear redness and irritation caused by the glare of the lights.

Steam fresh cabbage leaves in boiling water until they turn slightly limp. Drain and apply the warm leaves to your eyes for twenty minutes. If the leaves cool, replace them with warm ones.

Chamomile Sty Chaser

Brew chamomile tea (using the basic tea recipe). Strain and while still warm, use an eye dropper to bathe the eyes.

American-Indian Eye Wash

Pour boiling water over sesame leaves. Steep for at least five minutes, cool, and use the strained solution to bathe the eyes. Or you can soak a piece of gauze or clean cloth and apply it to your eyes. An alternate remedy is an eyewash made from yarrow leaves and flowers.

Eye Strain Wash

For tired, strained, reddened eyes, use this remedy twice a day. Combine one tablespoon each of the following dried herbs: goldenseal, eyebright, bayberry bark, red raspberry leaves.

Mix together well. Make a tea, using two teaspoons of herb mixture to one pint of pure water. Cool and strain. Do not use any single batch for more than one week.

Clear Eye Wash

Add one tablespoon of boric acid and one teaspoon of slippery elm powder to one pint of boiling water. Mix well. Cool and allow the ingredients to settle. Pour off the clear water or strain through clean gauze. Wash your eyes with this water as often as desired.

Clear Eye Wash II

Combine one teaspoon each of fennel, chamomile, and eyebright with three cups of boiling water. Cover until cool, then strain through a clean cloth. Wash your eyes with this solution as needed, up to every three to four hours.

Eyebright-Honey Lotion

Pour three-quarters pint of boiling water over one handful of eyebright flowers and leaves. Let stand until the mixture becomes lukewarm. Strain, then add three tablespoons of pure honey. Stir until dissolved. Soak cotton pads in the lotion, squeezing out excess liquid. Place the pads on your eyelids for fifteen to twenty minutes, dipping them into the solution as they become dry. You can also use an eye cup or dropper to wash your eyes with this mixture a few times a day.

A variation calls for substituting one and one-half cups of milk for the water.

Gypsy Eye Wash

Pour one pint of boiling water over four teaspoons of dried elder flowers. Cool and strain. Bottle and refrigerate. Use as needed.

Borage Eye Lotion

This refreshes eyes that are red, tired, and burning. Prepare a strong tea (doubling the amount of herbs) of fresh or dried borage leaves and flowers. Cool slightly, then dip cotton pads into the solution. Squeeze slightly to remove excess moisture, then place the pads over your eyes for at least fifteen minutes. If the pads dry out, dip them in the solution again.

Cucumber Toner

To reduce puffiness, place two one-quarter inch slices of refrigerated cucumber over your eyelids for twenty to thirty minutes.

Grit Remover

For grit, ashes, dirt, or any foreign particle that gets imbedded in the eye, simply place two drops of warmed olive oil directly on the eyeball. If the particle remains, see your doctor.

Castor Oil Drops

Be sure to use only a fresh bottle of castor oil for this to ensure that the oil has not turned rancid. Place one drop in the eyes near the lids. This relieves fatigued, inflamed eyes.

Vermont Honey Cure

Place a drop of pure honey in each eye to relieve strain. Or you can dissolve three tablespoons of honey in two cups of boiling water. Be sure the honey is completely dissolved. Cool and bathe your eyes several times a day. Or moisten cotton pads with the cold solution and use as compresses.

Pink Eye Cure

Brew elder blossom tea (according to the basic tea recipe). Cool and strain. Use as an eye wash until condition clears.

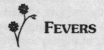 **FEVERS**

Onion Poultice

Slice an onion and place on your chest or put the slices against the soles of your feet and cover with white socks. This makes an effective fever cooler.

Fever Buster

Take one thumb-sized piece of ginger root, washed and peeled, and simmer in a cup or so of water heated to just before boiling point for two or three minutes. Add a pinch of cayenne pepper, one-quarter teaspoon of honey, and juice from one-half lemon. Drink as hot as possible, as quickly as possible. Ginger tea induces sweating; do not use in cases of extremely high fever.

Gypsy Elder Tea

Pour one cup of boiling water over two teaspoons of elder flowers. Steep for five to ten minutes. Drink to relieve the thirst that results from fevers. This tea is excellent for colds and flus; it also soothees nerves, induces sleep, and taken four times a day, helps relieve urinary problems. Some herbalists have used elder tea to clean the blood.

Mint Fever Tea

Steep one teaspoon of any mint leaves in hot water or put a few drops of peppermint oil in hot water. Sip slowly.

Fever Cooling Tea

Place one-quarter ounce of peppermint leaves and one-quarter ounce of elder flowers in a pottery or glass container. Boil two cups of water and pour over the herbs. Cover and steep for twenty minutes. Sweeten as desired. Strain and drink, then rest in bed or go to sleep. Use spearmint for children.

Sage Tea

Sage tea (using the basic tea recipe) has been proven in scientific studies to reduce fevers and night sweats.

Pomegranate Juice

The easiest way to get this fever-cooling juice is to buy it by the bottle at your health food store. Or you can juice it fresh in your juicer. Another option, particularly if you have a sore throat, is to eat the fruit raw, letting the juice trickle down your throat.

Tamarind Tea

Steep one ounce of tamarind pulp in one quart of water for one hour. Cool, then strain. Drink one-half cup of the liquid diluted with water, every three hours.

Quince Seed Tea

This pilgrim remedy was used to cool feverish colds. Brew a decoction (using the basic decoction recipe) of quince seeds. Cool, then strain. Take one cup, three or four times a day.

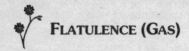

FLATULENCE (GAS)

Gas Buster Teas

Rosemary, or the seeds of either fennel, mustard, or anise all make teas that are useful in relieving gas. Simmer one table-spoon of the herb of your choice in one cup of boiling water for fifteen minutes. Mix with equal part of honey. Strain and take two tablespoons before each meal.

In the European-American herbal tradition, fennel tea—made from the boiled seeds—is traditionally used to soothe baby's colic, the discomfort caused by gas.

Slippery Elm Gas Relief Tea

Simmer one teaspoon of powdered or granulated slippery elm bark in two cups of water for twenty minutes. Strain and drink as needed. This tea also has a laxative effect, relieves vom-iting when the patient can't hold down anything else, and helps to heal stomach ulcers. It's especially beneficial for ba-bies and older people.

Fenugreek Tea

The tea made from these seeds soothes irritated bowel linings and helps to expel excess intestinal gas. Steep two teaspoons of fennel seeds in one cup of boiling water for five to ten minutes. Strain and drink as needed.

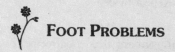 **FOOT PROBLEMS**

The feet are among the most important parts of the body to keep clean for overall health. Because of the weight and pressure borne by the bottoms of the feet, toxins expelled by the body tend to adhere there and clog the pores. Unless you keep your feet scrupulously clean, these toxins can be reabsorbed. To build up bone strength in your feet and toughen the soles, walk in dewy grass or in salt water as much as possible.

Gypsy Foot-Toughener

Soak pounded ivy leaves in vinegar for two days. Bathe your feet in the solution and rub well.

Foot Cooler

Another folk remedy from the Gypsies, this one helps prevent fatigue and overheating on long walks. It's awkward but effective. Line your socks (or shoes, if you're not wearing socks) with cabbage or marshmallow leaves. Or you can dust your toes with tobacco ash.

Hayflower and/or Oat Straw Foot Baths

Take three to five handfuls of hay, including the stalks, leaves, blossoms, and seeds. Pour one gallon of boiling water over the hay. Let the mixture cool to a comfortable warmth. Strain. Soak your feet for at least twenty minutes. This bath relieves excess sweating, helps heal open wounds, bruises, tumors, gout in the foot, ingrown nails, corns, blisters, and moves matter accumulated between the toes. Foot baths are best taken in alternating temperatures of warm and cold. Prepare enough to make two baths, one cold and one warm. Alternate ten minutes in the warm bath with one minute in the cold bath. Repeat twice.

Easy Callus Remover

Cut an onion bulb in half and place in a jar filled with strong wine vinegar. Steep for three hours or more. Bind the onion halves to the calluses, just before retiring at night. Repeat until all the layers of the calluses are removed.

Castor Oil

Apply castor oil often to calluses to soften them and relieve the pain. Frequent applications will also prevent the formation of calluses. A variation calls for mixing baking soda and castor oil, then applying in the same manner.

Yarrow Foot Bath

Add one cup of yarrow leaves and one tablespoon of salt to three quarts of hot water. Soak for at least twenty to thirty minutes. This will soften any corn, callus, or bunion and allow it to slough off.

For Athlete's Foot

Expose your toes to the air and sunlight as much as possible, and don't forget to wear a clean change of socks every day!

Onion Cure

Rub onion juice between the toes two or three times daily until the itching stops and the condition clears.

Red Clover Blossom Poultice
Boil one cup of red clover blossoms in one pint of water until thick. Apply directly to the affected areas. Cover, bind securely, and leave on overnight.

Apple Cider Vinegar
Washing your feet frequently in apple cider vinegar acidifies the area and discourages the growth of the fungus.

Vinegar-Alcohol Wash
Even more effective is to combine equal parts of cider vinegar and ethyl alcohol and sponge between the toes.

Powdered Alum Antiperspirant
This old country remedy calls for dusting powdered alum between the toes, on the soles of the feet, and inside your shoes.

Talcum Preventive
Borated talcum is a great prophylactic against athlete's foot and other fungi that love warm, moist, dark places. It can also arrest the fungus if caught in the early stages.

Shepherd's Remedy
Place small pieces of lambswool between the toes to absorb excess moisture. You can also dampen the wool with grated garlic or garlic juice to make a potent fungus fighter. Purchase lambswool in any store that stocks ballet dancer's supplies. In a pinch, absorbent cotton will do, especially when saturated with garlic.

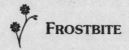

FROSTBITE

Aloe Vera

This is truly an amazing plant, able to heal burns *and* frostbite! In one study, after taking aspirin orally and applying aloe vera topically, all but one of forty-four patients suffering from frostbite had no major tissue loss—a remarkable result.

Mixed Oil Remedy

Mix together one ounce each of cold-pressed olive oil, peppermint oil, and ammonia. Rub on frostbitten hands and feet.

Cold Water Soak

Soak frostbitten hands and feet in cold water. Rub appendages but do not hold over direct heat.

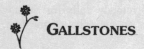 **GALLSTONES**

Olive Oil

Olive oil is a valuable preventative against gallstones. The oil causes strong healthy contractions of the gallbladder, helping it to empty itself of bile completely. It is therefore a great gallbladder tonic. In 1893, a doctor immersed a gallstone in pure olive oil and it lost sixty-eight percent of its weight in two days. Some healers recommend chasing six ounces of olive oil with six ounces of fresh lemon juice at night. Then lie on your right side for twenty minutes.

Parsley Juice

Take one teaspoon of fresh parsley juice every morning before breakfast.

Apple Juice Cleanse

Drink one gallon of pure apple juice each day, for two days in a row, spread out throughout the day. On the third day, drink one-half cup of cold-pressed, pure olive oil.

Gooseberry Tea

This bitter brew helps dissolve gallstones.

Chop coarsely one ounce of gooseberry leaves and roots. Simmer in one pint of water for twenty minutes. Drink one cup, three times a day.

Dandelion Decoction

Brew a strong tea from the leaves (doubling the amount of dandelion to water in the basic tea recipe). This tea contains many blood-purifying nutritive salts and it is also highly cleansing to the gallbladder and spleen.

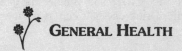

GENERAL HEALTH

In years past, mothers regularly administered bitter tonics to their families, especially during the changes in season. The herbs were often gathered by families and dried in their attics. Few of us live in areas where we can pick our own herbs, but we can do the next best thing. Instead of waiting for illness to strike, we can make use of the many tonic and health-boosting herbs available at health food stores and herb shops.

European Bitters for Americans

Bitters are liquors into which a bitter herb, root, or leaf has been crushed. The daily ingestion of bitters is to the herbalist as what an inoculation of vaccine is to Western conventional medicine. A small amount of bitters, however, will not create any side effects and could even be used to counteract many drug side effects.

Combine equal parts of the following powdered herbs: garlic, echinacea, goldenseal, and chaparral. Place the mixture in 00-size gelatin capsules and take two to four times a day. A couple of capsules could be taken each morning to maintain health and prevent disease. *Warning*: Do not take goldenseal for more than two weeks at a time. Do not use this tonic at all if you have high blood pressure. Use caution with garlic if you suffer from heartburn.

Gypsy Tonic

Mix together the following ingredients:

> ¼ ounce horseradish root
> 2 ounces celery root
> 1 ounce dandelion root

Place the ingredients in a saucepan with two pints of water and bring to a boil. Cover and simmer for twenty minutes. Strain and bottle. Drink one-half cup, two times a day.

Coconut

The meat or jelly of the young coconut contains a high percentage of sodium and is one of the best forms of potassium supplementation. The milk extracted from the hardened nut is used in cooking tasty Caribbean dishes.

Siberian Ginseng

Siberian ginseng, taken in capsule, tincture, tea form, or simply chewing on the root, is extremely beneficial for the glands. It strengthens the entire body, combats stress, and provides nutrition and tone. Ginseng, particularly the Siberian variety, contains extremely high levels of immune-system-boosting germanium. It is used by athletes for energy, stamina, stress reduction, and to combat high blood pressure, but ginseng is helpful for anyone.

Honey-Barley Gruel

This old folk remedy strengthens the entire body and heals the internal organs, cleans the blood, and invigorates the nerves. It's especially good for infants and invalids.

Bring four ounces of whole barley to a boil in just enough water to cover. Strain off. Pour one and one-half pints of water over the cleaned barley and simmer until the barley is soft, continually adding water to keep the amount at one and a half pints. Remove from heat and stir in three ounces of honey. Eat as desired.

Honey-Sunflower Iron Cordial

Place three-quarters cup of shelled sunflower seeds in a saucepan with six cups of water, one cup of chopped dates, one-half cup of raisins, one small orange, washed and quartered, and a one-quarter-inch piece of ginger root. Bring to a boil, then simmer for about half an hour. Remove from heat and steep until lukewarm. Strain. Stir in one cup of honey. Drink one-half cup, once or twice a day, or take as needed for energy.

Garlic-Honey-Lemon Lift

Combine one pound of peeled, pulped garlic with the juice of two dozen lemons. Heat to just below boiling point in a glass or enamel pot. Add one pound of honey. Heat again to just below boiling point. Cool slightly, pour mixture into jars, and cover loosely. When the mixture cools completely, screw the covers tightly and store in a lukewarm place for three weeks. Shake well and take one tablespoon in one-half cup of warm water before each evening meal. Or use as a salad dressing or pour over cooked vegetables.

Beet Liver Tonic

This tasty remedy cleanses and tones the liver. Express raw, whole beets in your juicer or scrape the beets and mix with a few drops of horseradish juice.

Cornsilk Tea

Valued also for its soothing effect on irritated bladders, this tea made from the silky hairs that line corn husks is also a good liver tonic, especially for those suffering from rheumatism. Boil one and one-half tablespoons of corn silk in one and one-half cups of water for ten minutes. Strain and drink hot, as needed. Sweeten with honey to taste.

Kola Nut

Available in capsules here, the kola nut is used by African mine workers to provide strength and endurance for work underground. **Warning**: the kola nut does contain caffeine.

Yellow Dock and Rocky Mountain Grape Root

Take two capsules, three times a day, of either herb to put iron in the blood if you are anemic or suffer from cold hands and feet. Yellow dock is full of minerals, especially iron, and it stimulates the liver and gallbladder secretions. Do not use yellow dock if you have urinary tract problems. It has a terrible taste, and is therefore best taken in capsule form.

Royal Jelly

Produced by the worker bees for the queen, this jelly sustains her through a life twenty times longer than the workers. Although all the ingredients are not known, royal jelly does contain B5 (calcium pantothenate), which has been shown to speed growth and increase resistance in laboratory animals. It also has antibacterial and antiviral properties against such organisms as streptococcus and staphylococcus. It accelerates formation of bone tissue, and when applied to wounds, promotes quicker healing. Take one vial daily.

Gentian Bitters

Gentian is used to make a simple bitter to stimulate the appetite, improve digestion, and as a general tonic. Dry the gentian roots, then cut up finely and add one-third cup to a bottle of brandy or lab-proof alcohol. Steep for one week, then strain. Put twenty to thirty drops in one-half glass of water three times daily to improve digestion and appetite. This is also helpful after meals to relieve a feeling of fullness as well as cramps.

For fatigue, some traditional herbalists recommended chewing a sugar cube infused with several drops of the bitter extract.

Blood-Building Teas

Use one teaspoon of walnut leaves, picked before the nuts form. Pour one cup of boiling water over leaves. Steep for five minutes and take one cup, three times a day.

Another traditional blood-builder is sassafras root. Make a decoction and brew according to the basic decoction recipe.

Wild Cherry Bark Body Builder

Add one ounce of wild cherry bark, the juice from one lemon, and two tablespoons of flax seeds to one quart of water. Bring to a boil and simmer for twenty minutes. Sweeten with honey to taste. Drink one-half cup, two times a day.

Amla Berry

Indian gooseberry, from the Himalayas, is rich in many antioxidants, and is reported to possess at least twenty times the vitamin C content of either acerola or rose hips. Take one capsule, three times a day, for endurance and energy.

Lycii Berries

Used in Oriental medicine, these berries help to promote cheerfulness and a long life, improve vitality and vision. Lycii is also considered a beneficial tonic for liver and kidneys, and it also helps to calm the nerves. These berries are delicious and can be added to food in much the same way one would add raisins. They are available at any Asian food store.

Dandelion Combination Tonic

Taken daily, this drink sharpens the senses, tones the arteries, and strengthens the liver. Combine two ounces of nettles with one ounce of dandelion root. Mix well. Pour one pint of boiling water over two or three tablespoons of the mixture. Steep for ten to twenty minutes. Add honey to taste. Use instead of coffee and tea.

Figs

Figs pack a great deal of nutrition—and calories—and are especially fortifying to those who are debilitated from long-term illness.

Dandelion Salad

This is a delicious and effective blood builder and tonic.

Chop one cup of dandelion leaves. Drip one teaspoon of honey over the leaves, followed by one teaspoon of olive oil and one-half teaspoon of lemon juice. Mix four teaspoonfuls of ground nuts in the salad.

Barberry Root

Taken in capsule form, one capsule three times a day, barberry is an effective tonic for the liver and gallbladder.

Nervous and Digestive System Toner

This tonic provides overall stimulation to the body, especially to the nervous system. It also promotes digestion and elimination.

Combine four ounces of prickly ash bark with one ounce

each of Irish moss and bayberry. Chop very finely. Take six ounces of the herb mixture and place in two quarts of distilled water. Let stand for two hours. Bring to a boil for thirty minutes. Strain while hot. Add two cups of blackstrap molasses and one cup of food grade glycerine. Boil for five minutes, stirring constantly. Cool, bottle, and cap well. Take three to four tablespoons three times a day.

Nettle Tea

Nettle is a versatile remedy used by Caribbean people, American Indians, East Indians, Pakistanis, and many others. Rich in mineral salts and vitamins, it is used to build blood in cases of anemia that have proved intractable to drugs. It promotes the flow of breast milk, aids in weight reduction, and alleviates kidney and bladder problems. Applied directly to the skin, it relieves the pains of rheumatism. It can be taken as a infusion by steeping two to three tablespoons of the leaves or the entire plant in one cup of boiling water for ten minutes. Take one cup, three times a day. You can make nettle juice by mixing it with an equal amount of water and taking one teaspoon, twice a day. You can also mix nettles with other vegetables or stew them in olive oil and onion—a perfect accompaniment to mashed potatoes.

American Indian Poplar Tonic

This remedy comes from the famous Indian herbalist John Lighthall. It was used in cases of general debility with poor digestion. Combine equal parts of the inner barks of the poplar tree, dogwood tree, and sarsaparilla root. Cut up finely and place in a quart bottle until it is half full. Add whiskey until full. Allow to sit for twelve hours. Take one tablespoon before each meal.

Sassafras Tonic

This tasty spring tonic was first made by American Indians, then adopted by the colonists. Use the bark of the root to make a decoction (using the basic decoction recipe.) You can use this drink as a substitute for coffee or tea, or you can take it three to four times daily as a blood purifier and general tonic.

Bowel Tonic

This formula from Dr. Christopher is effective for a variety of lower bowel problems. Its action is to regulate bowel movements and restore tone.

Combine two tablespoons of powdered cascara sagrada with one tablespoon each of powdered barberry root, rhubarb root, goldenseal, raspberry leaves, lobelia, and ginger root. Mix together well and place in 00-size gelatin capsules. Take two capsules, two or three times a day. Use this remedy for two weeks, then take one week off, two weeks on, one week off, etc. Goldenseal root is not meant for continuous, long-term use. Do not use if you have high blood pressure.

Liver Tonic

This tonic is helpful in detoxifying the liver, whether diet or disease has caused the problem.

Combine two ounces each of Oregon grape root, wild yam root, and dandelion root with one-half ounce licorice root. Chop the roots finely. Bring two quarts of distilled water to a boil. Add the herb mixture and cook over a low heat for forty-five minutes to an hour. Strain and refrigerate. Take two warm tablespoons, three or four times a day, at least one-half hour before meals.

A Peachy Tonic

Peaches contain large quantities of iron, which makes them a great tonic for "tired blood." American Indians used apricots, also rich in iron and other vitamins, for the same reason. They brewed a decoction from the roots (using the basic decoction recipe) for anemic children. Elderly people drank a tea made from the leaves (using the basic tea recipe).

Overall Strengthening Tonic

This is effective for conditions of weakness, especially in women.

Combine the following herbs:

> 8 ounces alfalfa
> 2 ounces burdock root
> 1 ounce ginseng
> 1 ounce dong quai

Use four ounces of herb mixture per quart of water. Simmer for one hour. Strain. Return the liquid to the pot and add equal parts of a mixture of honey and barley malt syrup. Keep on low heat for five minutes, stirring to blend thoroughly. Take two tablespoons, three times a day, before meals. Do not use if you have yeast infections or candidiasis.

Pumpkin Tonic

Pumpkin is an easily digestible tonic food, especially when eaten raw and grated. It is packed with nutrients and strengthening to the system. You can brew a tea from the flowers, using three blossoms to one-half pint of boiling water. You can eat the meat in virtually any form—baked, steamed, sauteed, or raw—in pies, puddings, cakes, and soups. Or you can eat the most nutritious part—the seeds. These seeds pack a range of healing properties, making them effective remedies against such diverse ailments as malaria and high cholesterol. Full of vitamins, minerals, and protein, pumpkin seeds strengthen teeth and gums and help to prevent decay. Their high vitamin A and B2 content helps correct night blindness.

Catnip-Lemon Tea

Though catnip is known for its ability to soothe the nerves and stomach, when combined with lemon, it has tonic qualities. Brew a tea using two teaspoons of dried herb to one cup of water. Steep for five to ten minutes, then add lemon and honey to taste.

Chamomile-Lime-Licorice Tonic

Pour one pint of boiling water over one teaspoon each of licorice root powder, chamomile flowers, and lime flowers. Cover and steep for five minutes. Strain and drink as desired.

Female Tonic Tea

Wash and soak three tablespoons of juniper berries in cold water for fifteen minutes. Drain and simmer for thirty minutes in three cups of water. Strain out the berries. Place one teaspoon each of chamomile flowers and licorice powder in container. Reheat the juniper water to boiling and pour over the herb mixture. Cover and steep for five minutes. Strain and divide the liquid into four parts, each of which should be one-half cupful. Take one-half cup, four times a day.

Chamomile Sugar

This pep-up treat also helps to relieve coughs and hoarseness.

Make chamomile oil by mixing one and one-half pints of safflower oil with three ounces of dried chamomile leaves. Simmer in a glass or stainless steel saucepan for forty minutes. Remove from heat and let stand overnight. Strain and bottle.

Combine the chamomile oil with equal parts date sugar, and take by the tablespoonful as needed.

Borage Juice

This is best made with a vegetable juicer. Simply feed the fresh, washed leaves into the machine. If you are using a blender, break up the leaves a bit and blend them with enough water to make juice. This tasty, mineral-rich juice can be stored in the refrigerator or freezer and added to summer and holiday drinks.

Borage Candies

This treat is great for youngsters of all ages—delicious and health-promoting.

Mix together one beaten egg white and one tablespoon of orange juice. Beat until the mixture is fluffy, then dip fresh, opened borage flowers into the mixture, coating them thoroughly. Dust confectioner's sugar over each flower. Place between layers of wax paper and refrigerate or freeze for future use. Do not use if you have candidiasis or other yeast infections.

You can do the same with violets and rose petals.

Honeysuckle Bark Tea

This tea is said to strengthen the heart, decrease fluid retention, and reduce swollen lymph glands.

Make a decoction (using the basic decoction recipe) with honeysuckle bark. Drink one cup, three times a day.

Quick Energy Boosts

Take one capsule, three times a day, of any one of the following: Siberian ginseng, ground poppy or chia (from sage) seeds. The body cannot assimilate seeds in their whole form. Steep one teaspoon of chia seeds for twelve hours in a cold glass of water. Then sweeten the mucilaginous drink with honey and take in the morning. Or you can grind the seeds and sprinkle them over salads, stir them into soups, or use them with butter as a spread.

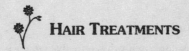 **HAIR TREATMENTS**

Healthy Scalp Prescription

Brew a strong tea of equal parts dried nettles, rosemary, comfrey, and witch hazel leaves. Add one-half ounce (about one handful) of the herbs to two cups of water. Bring to a boil in a covered pot and remove from stove immediately. Let it sit overnight. After shampooing and rinsing your hair with plain water, use the herbal tea as a final rinse. The herbal combination is soothing, astringent, and antiseptic. If your scalp problem is fungal or bacterial, add one drop of tea tree oil to the brew just before you rinse your hair.

Hair Restorer

Rub aloe vera gel into your scalp. Leave on overnight and shampoo in the morning. It is said that this treatment remedies baldness.

Falling Hair Cure

Crush well one-half cup of rosemary leaves and steep in one pint of pure alcohol for one week. Rub the scalp with this solution twice a day as a treatment for falling hair.

Sage Hair Conditioner

This is a great conditioner to darken gray hair. Place two heaping tablespoons of sage and two tablespoons of ordinary tea in one pint of boiling water. Cover and heat slowly in an oven for two hours. The longer it heats, the darker the mixture becomes. Strain and add a tablespoon of brandy or vodka to preserve, unless you are using it up within the next few days. Rub the cold infusion into your hair roots nightly.

Baldness Cure

No guarantees come with this remedy, which is supposed to work if the hair roots are still alive! Mix one ounce of onion juice with one ounce of crude cod liver oil and one-half ounce of raw egg yolk. Beat together thoroughly and apply to your scalp once a week. You can also rub your scalp with a fresh onion slice once or twice daily.

Dandruff Remedies

The worst thing you can do is use a commercial dandruff shampoo. These preparations remove the dandruff initially, but it seems to come back even worse!

Marigold and Nettle Rinse
Make a strong tea (two teaspoons per one cup of water) with marigold and nettles. Use as the final rinse whenever you wash your hair.

Herbal Oil Dandruff Chaser
Dilute one teaspoon each of the essential oils of cedarwood, lavender, and rosemary in one cup of a vegetable oil base, such as coconut or almond oil, and massage into the scalp.

Rosemary Tea Rinse
Combine rosemary tea with borax and allow the mixture to cool for an effective hair rinse that cleanses the scalp and helps to rid it of dandruff. This remedy is said to prevent premature baldness.

Another formula specific against dandruff and baldness is to combine one ounce each of rosemary and sage and infuse them in one pint of hot water for twenty-four hours. Strain and use as a final rinse when you wash your hair.

Nettle-Vinegar Rinse
Steep one-quarter cup of dried nettles in one cup of boiling water. Cool and add one-quarter cup of cider vinegar. Massage into your scalp twice daily.

Apple Cider Vinegar Rinse
This old-fashioned remedy is also effective. Warm the vinegar, pour it on, then let it set for an hour before washing it out.

The following herbs can be added to your shampoo to increase its desired effects.

Balm—stimulates healthy hair growth, and gives a soothing effect.

Betaine—conditions and neutralizes negatively charged hair so that it is not unkempt or flyaway.

Birch—antiseptic and astringent, kills bacteria, neutralizes irritants, and strengthens tissues.

Clover—emollient and bactericide.

Coltsfoot—soothes delicate, easily inflamed scalp.

Fennel—calming and antiseptic.

Henna—gives hair shine, smoothes the hair shaft, untangles hair.

Hops—softens, promotes healthy cell growth, a natural preservative.

Horsetail—stimulates growth and combats dandruff.

Mistletoe—stimulates the immune system.

Nettle—counterirritant, calms and stimulates metabolism.

Panthenol—protects the hair, makes it flexible.

Rosemary—conditions, stimulates circulation of blood to the scalp.

Yarrow—antiinflammatory, antiseptic, stimulates growth, fights dandruff and other unhealthy scalp conditions.

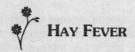 **Hay Fever**

Onion Drink

Juice an onion and mix with an equal part of water. Take one teaspoon every three minutes until symptoms subside.

Hay Fever Reliever

This old recipe is said to relieve the local irritation that accompanies bouts of hay fever. Combine the following tinctures:

> ½ ounce wood betony
> 1 ounce yarrow
> ¾ ounce euphrasia
> 10 drops of capsicum

Combine with eight ounces of water. Take three table-spoons in one-half cup of water, three times a day.

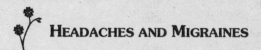

HEADACHES AND MIGRAINES

It used to be popular to say that ninety percent of headaches and migraines are caused by nervous tension. While techniques such as head and neck massage, acupuncture and acupressure, guided meditation, progressive relaxation, and biofeedback are helpful in many cases, studies indicate that other factors such as diet, allergies, hormone imbalances and hormone replacement therapy, as well as environmental pollutants, may be the root causes of headaches and migraines. The following remedies offer relief, but if you suffer from chronic headaches or migraines, consult your doctor.

Vinegar Headache Cure

Mix together equal parts of vinegar and water and inhale the fumes. Or you can refrigerate the solution and sponge your forehead, the back of your neck, temples and under your chin. Let it dry.

Vinegar and Brown Bag Headache Cure

A variation of the above remedy involves a plain brown bag. Cut strips wide and long enough to cover your forehead and temples. Soak them in vinegar and then lie down, placing the strips on top of each other and covering your forehead and temples. Let them dry, molding themselves onto your upper face. Wear them all day.

Rosemary Tea

This versatile tea helps to relieve headaches and nervous tension. It is also effective for colic and colds.

Primrose Tea

Brew a tea with dried primrose leaves and flowers (slightly stronger than the basic tea recipe). Steep for fifteen to twenty minutes, sweeten with honey to taste.

Lavender Tea

For nervous headaches and stomachs, brew fresh or dried lavender flowers (using the basic tea recipe). Take as needed. If the taste is too powerful, mix with chamomile, hops, lemon balm, or any other nervine herbs.

Sinus Headache Tea

This tea will clear up any respiratory congestion that is causing a headache. Use it both as a drink and as an inhalant steam. Brew equal parts of wild cherry bark, eucalyptus, and mullein, with licorice root to improve the taste. Stand over the herbs as they simmer on the stove with a towel over your head as a hood and breathe in the vapors. Drink up to three or four cups a day.

Wood Betony Tea

Make a tea (using the basic tea recipe) by steeping one ounce of the herb in one pint of boiling water for ten minutes. Take as often as needed to relieve headaches due to nervous tension.

Onion Poultice

This one's messy but effective in two hours! Pulp three or four onions. Salt generously and mix with olive oil. Spread the mixture on a cloth and bind it to the head.

Hops Tea

This is said to relieve headaches brought on by tension and other nervous conditions. Brew a tea (using the basic tea recipe) and take a small cupful every two or three hours.

Hops Tonic Water

This drink soothes headaches caused by nervous stomachs, induces sleep, calms frazzled nerves, and is a general strengthening tonic for the body.

Brew one cup of hops tea (using the basic tea recipe) and combine with an equal part of tonic (also known as quinine) water. Drink as needed.

Herbal Teas

Pour boiling water over catnip, peppermint, or sage and brew for three to five minutes for a calming drink.

Feverfew

Take either 25 mg. of the freeze-dried leaves daily on an empty stomach for three months, or take it as a tincture, thirty drops, twice a day, or one capsule, three times a day. Supporting herbs, such as skullcap and chamomile, can also be taken in tea form.

Combination Tea

Mix together equal parts of skullcap, valerian, rosemary, chamomile, and peppermint. Make a tea (using the basic decoction formula). Take one-half cup every hour until the pain dissipates.

Nervous Stomach Headache Tea

This tea works beautifully for headaches caused by nervous stomachs.

Mix together one-third teaspoon each of chamomile, mint, and catnip. Pour one cup of boiling water over the herb mixture. Steep for five to ten minutes, then strain. Take up to one cup, three or four times a day, or as needed.

Migraines and Tightness of Scalp

This type of headache can be caused by a reaction to an allergen, a possibility that should be checked out with your doctor or health caretaker.

Rosemary Combination Migraine Tea
Combine the following:

> 2 ounces of wood betony
> 1 ounce of rosemary
> 1 ounce of skullcap

Mix thoroughly and place one-quarter of the mixture in one pint of cold water. Bring to a boil and simmer for two minutes. Strain and leave until cold. Drink one-half cup, three times a day. If insomnia is involved, drink an extra dose, hot, at bedtime.

Vinegar-Hops Compress
Mix two tablespoons of vinegar with two cups of hops tea. Soak a clean cloth or gauze in the solution. Apply while still warm to the forehead. Drink a cup of hops tea.

Gypsy Nettle Cure
Boil one tablespoon of nettles in one pint of milk for fifteen minutes. Drink as needed to relieve the head pain and the vomiting that often accompanies migraines.

Essential Oil Rub

Blend together one drop of peppermint oil, three drops of lavender oil, and one drop of a cold-pressed vegetable oil. Beginning at the temples and working your way down to the base of the skull, massage your head with this oil in slow, circular motions away from the face. This induces a state of relaxation that can bring effective relief.

Herbal Inhalations

This is a popular remedy among country folk. Among the herbs sniffed to quell migraine headaches are crushed lemon verbena leaves, fresh hops, bruised dill or dill seed, cloves, sage, peppermint, spearmint, dried orange or lemon peels, betony rose leaves, lavender buds, and violets. Or you can use herbal oils made from any of the above.

Rosemary Spirits

Make a tincture (using the basic tincture recipe) of rosemary leaves and tops. As soon as a headache begins, hold the bottle containing rosemary spirits close to the nostrils and inhale the fumes. In addition, rub a few drops of this remedy on the temples, forehead, veins of the neck, and behind the ears.

American Indian Elder Cure

The Choctaw Indians pounded elder leaves and mixed them with salt to make a compress. Place the mixture in a clean cloth or gauze and tape securely to your forehead.

American Indian Cedar Cure

Soak small twigs of cedar in water until they soften. Bind them to your forehead.

White Rose Cure

Fill a quart jar with closely packed white rose petals. Pour in 70 percent rubbing alcohol until the jar is full. Let the jar stand uncovered in the sun all day, or by the pilot light of your stove. If the alcohol evaporates, fill the jar again. At the end of the day, cover the jar and refrigerate. Whenever you have a headache, sponge your forehead, temples, the back of your neck, and under your chin. Or soak a cloth and apply it as a compress to your forehead and temples.

Mustard Footbath

This helps to draw circulation away from the head and towards the lower extremities. Place one tablespoon of dried mustard in boiling water. When it has cooled sufficiently, soak your legs and feet in the hot solution for as long as possible. The same effect can be achieved with a hot ginger foot bath.

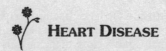

HEART DISEASE

Heart disease is one health problem that has shown improvement in recent years. Overall, more and more Americans are quitting smoking, lowering the amount of fat in their diets, lowering their serum cholesterol, and taking supplements to increase their health. Studies indicate that certain nutritional substances can be of great benefit to your heart.

Cuppa Tea

A few cups of tea a day may be supportive of heart health and function. Flavenoids—an antioxidant found in fruits and vegetables as well as in tea and wine—lessen the tendency of blood to form clots in the arteries that supply the heart muscle. Recent research indicates that the more flavenoids consumed, the lower the risk of heart attack. Ordinary tea contains a rich supply of flavenoids.

Green tea is even more effective. Many heart attacks are caused by the aggregation of blood platelets, which form blood clots that accumulate as plaque on artery walls and block the flow of blood through coronary arteries. Green tea inhibits the production of platelet activity factor, a cause of blood "clumping." Green tea also reduces high blood pressure, another heart disease risk factor. Prescription drugs combat high blood pressure by inhibiting the formation of an enzyme called angiotension-converting enzyme (ACE), which is secreted by the kidneys and causes blood vessel constriction. Green tea also limits the formation of ACE.

Hawthorn Berry

For ages, this herb was eaten in large quantities by American Indians to protect against heart attack. An extremely safe herb, hawthorn can be used as a long-term heart tonic without side effects. Its effect is sustained, countering degenerative, age-related changes in the heart muscles, preventing arrhythmias, reducing cardiac asthma and edema, and regulating the heart beat. It can be used in teas (using the basic tea formula), or a tincture (twenty to forty drops twice daily), or made into jellies and jams.

Heart Strengthening Tip

A folk healer once advised that chewing on dried currants and raisins throughout the day and eating the tops of rosemary right after breakfast are strengthening to the heart.

A Clove a Day

In recent years, research has uncovered garlic's cholesterol-lowering powers. High blood cholesterol levels play a major role in heart disease, including atherosclerosis, or narrowing of the arteries, which leads to heart attacks and strokes. Participants in studies who took between 600 to 1,000 mg. of garlic in tablet or powder or extract form a day, showed an average of 9 percent lowered cholesterol levels. Or you can take one-half to one whole garlic clove a day.

Onion

Onions have a cleansing effect on the arteries, decreasing blood cholesterol levels and fighting off excessive platelet aggregation.

Alfalfa

This humble grain contains a mystery agent that lowers cholesterol levels. The seeds may raise the ratio of high-density lipoproteins (HDL) to low-density lipoproteins (LDL). Alfalfa sprouts and ground seeds make a delicious garnish for salads and a welcome addition to sandwiches. Try two teaspoons of ground alfalfa seeds per meal.

Yogurt

Yogurt is another mysterious cholesterol combatant. Research shows that it can lower blood cholesterol, yet an equal amount of unfermented milk is completely ineffective.

Cayenne Pepper (Capsicum)

This herb is a pure and potent stimulant. It goes to work so rapidly that its action begins when it's held in the mouth a short time. Cayenne pepper is wonderful for the circulatory system, restoring elasticity to the blood vessels and equalizing the flow of blood throughout the body. It also helps dissolve blood clots when they're still small and helps to rebuild the mucus lining of the stomach and heal intestinal ulcers. Take one capsule, three times a day.

Fenugreek Tea

This wonderful tea (using the basic decoction recipe) contains choline, a substance known to soften and dissolve cholesterol that accumulates on the walls of blood vessels and in the liver. Drink one cup, three times a day, or as often as desired.

Artery Clearing and Conditioning Tonic

Clogged arteries and high cholesterol levels contribute to heart disease. The artery-clearing tonic prevents and helps to cure this dangerous condition.

Dissolve two teaspoons of honey, one tablespoon of lecithin granules, and two teaspoons of safflower oil in one cup of fenugreek tea. Drink one cup a day to prevent clogged arteries; drink two or three a day if your arteries are already clogged.

Herbal Heartbeat Regulator

Mix together one teaspoon each of the following powdered herbs: black cohosh, scullcap, valerian root, lobelia root, and cayenne. Steep in one pint of boiling water for at least ten minutes. Drink one to two cups a day, at least one-half hour before meals.

Herbal Blood Thinners

Teas made from either sassafras, burdock, or red clover (using the basic tea or decoctionr recipe) thin and cleanse the blood.

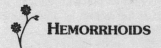

HEMORRHOIDS

Pain relief can be obtained simply by wiping the rectum with toilet paper or cotton pads soaked in warm water after each bowel movement. Then use dry toilet paper or cotton. Use only no-fragrance, no-dye toilet paper.

Witch Hazel Pads

Cotton pads saturated with witch hazel stop the itching and bleeding associated with hemorrhoids. Apply witch hazel not only after bowel movements but several times throughout the day to help shrink swollen veins. You can also leave the witch-hazel-soaked pad on the affected area for ten to fifteen minutes whenever possible.

Witch Hazel–Herb Pads

Combine the following herbs:

> 1 ounce witch hazel leaves
> ½ ounce bayberry bark
> ½ ounce goldenseal

Mix with two pints of boiling water and simmer for twenty to thirty minutes. Add one pint of glycerine. Fill a small medicine dropper and insert into the rectum three times a day.

Alum Sitz Bath

Mix one pound of alum into a sitz bath of hot water. Sit until the water cools.

Comfrey Root Ointment

Mix powdered comfrey root with enough water to make a paste. Apply inside the rectum as often as needed.

Comfrey Mixed Poultice

Mix together equal parts of comfrey, marigold, malva, red clover, burdock, elder, and yellow dock. Add enough olive oil to make a paste. Apply inside the rectum. Repeat until relief is obtained.

Olive Oil

After a bowel movement, clean the anus and then apply olive oil inside the rectum.

Yarrow Tea

Brew this tea by steeping two tablespoons in one cup of boiling water for fifteen minutes, then straining. Apply inside the rectum.

Hot/Cold Compresses

Place a washcloth in very hot water and another washcloth in ice water. Apply the hot cloth for three minutes, then apply the cold cloth for thirty seconds. Repeat twice.

Combination Tea

Combine the following herbs:

> 2 ounces dandelion root
> 1 ounce chicory root
> 1 ounce cascara
> sagrada
> ½ ounce licorice

Chop finely and mix two ounces with two pints of water to make a decoction. Drink one-half cup of tea, two or three times a day.

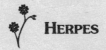 **HERPES**

Apple Slices

Apply a slice of yellow apple to the sore as often as necessary.

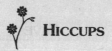 **HICCUPS**

Chamomile Oil

This variation on breathing into a paper bag is even more effective. Place a drop or two of chamomile oil in the bottom of the bag. Hold the opening of the bag over your mouth and nose. Breath deeply through your nose, in and out, until the hiccups stop.

Blue Cohosh Tea

Prepare a tea from either blue cohosh or black cohosh (using the basic tea recipe) or place ten to fifteen drops of either tincture in one-half cup of warm water. Drink as needed.

Pineapple Remedy

Holding your breath, take a few swallows of canned pineapple juice. Repeat once an hour, until relief is obtained.

Tartar Remedy

Mix together one-third teaspoon of cream of tartar and eight ounces of warm water. Take two tablespoons on an empty stomach.

Peanut Butter Remedy

Take one teaspoon of peanut butter. Repeat a few times until relief is obtained.

HIVES

Baking Soda Poultice

Make a paste with water and baking soda. Apply to affected area. This will relieve the itching and smooth out the bumps.

Dandelion Combination

Combine the following:

>1 ounce of nettles
>1 ounce of yarrow
>¼ ounce of goldenseal
>2 ounces of dandelion root

Simmer for twenty to thirty minutes in two pints of water. Take one tablespoon every four hours. You can also take a bath in this water to soothe any skin irritation.

Nettle Tincture

Apply five-drop doses of nettle tincture four or five times daily. Or you can prepare a nettle leaf decoction (using the basic decoction recipe) and let it boil down to a paste. Cool and rub the paste on affected areas. Drink a cup of nettle leaf tea (using the basic tea recipe) at the same time.

Mulberry All-Purpose Mash

Pulverize a handful of mulberries in the blender at low speed, until they form a coarse mash. Use as a poultice to remedy a variety of skin conditions, including hives, acne, ringworm, and impetigo.

Catnip Wash

Steep two tablespoons of bruised catnip leaves in one cup of
boiling water for ten minutes. Cool, strain, and apply to hives.

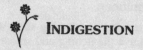

INDIGESTION

Mint Tea

Either peppermint or spearmint tea will settle queasy stomachs and make a wonderful conclusion to any meal. They also
relieve vomiting. Peppermint should not be used if you have
heartburn. Spearmint is more soothing and better for children
and babies. Use the basic tea recipe.

Chamomile Tea

Use the basic tea recipe. Though chamomile tea also stimulates digestive functions and aids in acid production, unlike
most herbs with similar functions, it does not taste bitter.

Papaya

Wherever this delicious fruit grows, the native inhabitants use
its juice or leaves to tenderize meats and eat the unripened
fruit to cure indigestion. Papaya contains papain, an enzyme
also secreted in the stomach to break down all types of foods
so that they can be easily digested. Eat freely, especially if
you have difficulty digesting meats.One-half cup of papaya
juice after each meal supplies sluggish tummies with helpful
digestive enzymes.You can also take papaya supplements.

Rosemary Tea

This tea (using the basic tea recipe) stimulates digestion,
makes a good female tonic, soothes the digestive tract, pro-

vides antiseptic and astringent effects, and helps eliminate excess mucus.

Juniper Berry Tea

A mild juniper berry tea (made according to the basic tea recipe) is a good remedy for colicky infants.

Hops

Pour one cup of boiling water over one teaspoon of hops. Steep for five minutes. Drink before meals and just before bedtime to soothe a nervous stomach.

Goldenrod Tea

This is another old Gypsy cure. Make a decoction (using the basic decoction recipe) from goldenrod leaves. Take one cup, three times a day, as an overall digestive tract strengthener.

Stomach Relief

Combine the following:

> 1 ounce gentian
> 1 ounce valerian
> 2 ounces roasted dandelion powder
> ½ teaspoon cayenne

Mix well. Pour one pint of boiling water over the herbs. Cool, strain, and bottle for use. Take one-half cup, three times a day, to relieve upset stomachs, especially when complicated by diseases of the liver, spleen, or pancreas.

Dandelion Tea

This is a favorite American Indian remedy. Brew a tea with the leaves and flowers (using the basic tea recipe). To heal

chronic liver and indigestion problems, drink one-half cup,
three times a day. (This tea also helps heal chronic kidney
problems, and dandelion's high iron content makes it an excellent food for the anemic.)

Heartburn Cure

Four ounces of goat's milk, taken three times a day, is a good
remedy for excessive belching and heartburn.

Digestive Wine

Combine one part each of dandelion root, calamus root, gentian, angelica, and valerian with one-half part ginger root and
one pint of good dry wine. Let it stand for two weeks, shaking
daily. Take one teaspoon before and after meals.

Valerian Root

Drop twenty to thirty drops of the tincture (using the basic
tincture recipe or purchased at a health food store) in one-
half cup of water to strengthen digestion, and drink before or
after meals. It speeds up digestion and perks up sluggish appetites.

Carrot and Potato Stomach Soother

Mash one cooked carrot with one cooked potato. Add a drop
of olive oil and a pinch of salt. Eat as a meal.

Acidity Neutralizing Drink

This is much better for you than downing any of the patented
acid stomach relievers on the market.
    Combine one large lemon and one cup of chopped celery
leaves with one pint of cold water. Mix thoroughly in the
blender. Add a little more water and honey to taste.

Digestive Fruit Soup

This delicious fruit soup cleanses and tones the entire digestive tract.

Soak two cups of raisins and two cups of prunes overnight in four quarts of water. In the morning, add one cup of unsweetened grape juice and two peeled and sliced lemons. Sweeten with honey to taste, and take as desired.

Orange Peel Tea

Organic orange peel, dried and steeped as a tea, relieves sluggish digestion.

Fennel

If your meal leaves you with that "stuffed" feeling, try chewing a few fennel seeds as a tasty digestive aid. In some parts of Asia and India, fennel seeds are traditionally offered after meals. The aromatic oils contained in fennel seeds stimulate the flow of digestive fluids and relieve gas pains by making you burp. Fennel also soothes the mucosa of the digestive tract and helps expel gas. It also relieves diarrhea by modifying bacteria in the small intestine.

Lightly toasting fennel seeds improves their flavor. Roast the seeds in a dry skillet for a minute or two over medium heat, stirring constantly to prevent burning. Let the seeds cool completely before storing them in a covered glass jar. If you prefer, fennel seeds can be made into a tea that will aid digestion. Pour one cup of boiling water over one teaspoon of fennel seeds. Cover and let steep for ten minutes before drinking. Fennel seeds can also be boiled in milk. Boil two teaspoons of the seeds in one cup of milk, turn off heat, strain, and drink the milk warm before meals, two to three times a day.

Digestive Paste

This paste is a natural antihistamine, stimulating digestion, and preventing the formation of excess mucus. Mix together equal parts of the following powdered herbs: black pepper, pippli pepper, and ginger. Mix with enough honey to form a paste. Take one teaspoon before meals.

Slippery Elm Tea

For a wonderfully soothing tea to the entire digestive tract, mix two teaspoons of slippery elm powder in one-half cup of cold water. Place in the blender for ten seconds. Add one pint of boiling water and stir well. Flavor with a little lemon juice or cinnamon.

Slippery Elm Porridge

Heat one-half pint of milk and sprinkle in one-half to one teaspoon of powdered slippery elm. Put in blender and mix thoroughly. Bring to a boil and stir the mixture until it thickens. Sweeten with honey to taste. Some people like to beat in one egg with the powdered bark, then pour boiling milk over the mixture and sweeten to taste.

Post-Mealtime Indigestion Capsules

If an upset stomach follows every meal take one capsule *each* of powdered goldenseal and cayenne pepper with one cup of warm water, one-half hour before meals, to cleanse the digestive tract.

Stomach Flu Relief

Combine equal parts of the following powdered herbs: goldenseal, slippery elm, cinnamon, and cayenne pepper. Mix thoroughly. Fill 00-size gelatin capsules. Take one capsule with one-half glass of warm water before meals or as needed. One dose is usually enough, but you can take this for a few days, if necessary. If you are vomiting, do not use this remedy because the bitter taste of the goldenseal will be repeated.

Anti-Vomiting Teas

Taken in capsule or tea forms, any of the following herbs will stop vomiting caused by a viral infection: cinnamon, clove, peach leaf, catnip, peppermint, spearmint, chamomile.

Barley Water

Place one cup barley in a strainer, and rinse well with cold water. Add barley to two quarts water in a pot. Bring to a boil and simmer fifteen minutes. Strain the water. Sip in small amounts to combat vomiting and ease a troubled tummy. This soothing drink is especially helpful for babies and older people, as well as heavily sedated postoperative patients whose normal enzyme production is low.

Irish Moss

A favorite drink among Caribbean-Americans, Irish moss is a seaweed that has nutritive properties and a soothing effect similar to barley water. Use the same proportions and cook as you do barley water.

Aloe Vera Juice

Aloe vera juice peps up sluggish digestions, soothes and helps restore the mucus lining of the digestive tract, and promotes better assimilation of nutrients. Drink one quart daily—before meals if the digestive tract is irritated, after meals if digestion is simply sluggish. Children can take one tablespoon diluted in six ounces of water up to three times daily.

Jamaican Pimento Liqueur

This popular cordial among country folk in Jamaica settles upset stomachs and relieves diarrhea.

Combine the following:

1½ quarts ripe pimento berries
4 pounds sugar
2 quarts water
1 quart rum
¾ pound cinnamon sticks
1 pint lime juice

Place the berries in the rum and lime juice for three days. Crack the cinnamon and boil in two quarts of water. Strain and boil with four pounds of sugar for about ten minutes. Squeeze out the berries, and add the sugar-cinnamon syrup when cold. Strain through clean muslin cloth and bottle. Take as needed.

Basil Tea

Brew (using the basic tea recipe). Take one cup, three times a day, to cure indigestion, calm the nerves, and relieve headaches.

Flax Seed

This is a wonderful herb for the entire digestive tract, especially the lower tract. Soak one tablespoon in one cup of water overnight, then bring to a boil and simmer ten minutes. Strain and sip.

Honeysuckle Tea

This tea is especially beneficial to those suffering chronic indigestion due to a liver and/or spleen disorder.

Mix three-quarters cup of leaves and one-quarter cup of blossoms in one pint of water. Simmer for ten minutes. Drink one cup, two times a day, before meals.

Chamomile-Allspice

Prepare a cup of chamomile (using the basic tea recipe). Add one-eighth teaspoon of ground allspice. Take as needed.

Nerves, Headache, and Digestive Tonic

This is especially effective for those with a poor hydrochloric acid output (as is the case with vegetarians returning to a diet that includes meats).

Place one pound of finely chopped celery stalks and leaves in a jar. Bring two pints of cider vinegar to a boil and remove from the burner. Stir in one tablespoon of dried kelp flakes (available at your health food store or herb store). Pour over the celery. Cover tightly. Take two teaspoons in one-half cup of either hot or cold water, two or three times a day, before meals.

Ginger-Mint

Prepare one cup of ginger root tea (using the basic decoction recipe) and one cup of mint tea (using the basic tea recipe) and combine them. Or you can add one-eighth teaspoon of powdered ginger to a cup of mint tea. Add lemon and honey to taste, and take as needed.

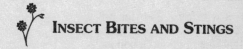

INSECT BITES AND STINGS

There are many excellent home remedies for insect bites and stings. Use whichever of the following is most convenient.

Toothpaste

Yep! Apply a little dab of ordinary toothpaste to a mosquito bite to take out the itch pronto. (This also works on pimples.)

Juniper Berry Solution

Brew a decoction of juniper berries. Cool, then strain and apply to the bite or sting or any poisonous insect. Let dry and repeat as needed.

Papaya Poultice

If fresh papaya is available, the flesh makes a great meat tenderizer, including your own! Simply take a slice of the fruit and bind it to the bite.

Meat Tenderizer

Dissolve one-quarter teaspoon of any meat tenderizer in one teaspoon of water. Rub into the skin around the bite or sting.

Cornstarch-Lemon Poultice

Make a paste from cornstarch and lemon juice or witch hazel. Apply to the mosquito bite.

Bee Sting Soother

Pour cold water into a pot, add a one-half cup of baking soda and stir. Add a tray of ice cubes. Soak the affected limb in the pot and the pain should stop almost instantaneously.

Onion Relief

Apply a freshly cut slice of onion to the sting. Hold or tape it in place.

Oatmeal Soak

If your body is covered with bites, dump a box of oatmeal and/or quick starch into a tub of water and soak for at least twenty minutes. If you can't get to a bathtub, make a paste of the oatmeal and apply to affected areas.

Tobacco Soother

Moisten tobacco and apply it to the bite. If you can get a tobacco leaf, that's even better.

Honey Soother

Dab generous amounts of honey or wheat germ oil on the sting, then apply ice or place the affected area in a pot of cold water and ice.

Honey-Soda Relief

Mix honey with enough baking soda to make a salve that will stick to the skin. Cover the insect bite or sting with a thick coat and let it dry. A variation calls for a paste made from baking soda and cider vinegar.

Plantain Healer

Plantain leaf is also helpful, both for mosquito bites and insect stings. Tear off a few leaves and bruise or break them. Heat the bruised leaves with a match until they wilt. Squeeze out the juice and apply to the sting or bite. The Chippewa Indians chopped up plantain roots and leaves to make a poultice for poisonous reptile bites.

Basil Water

Prepare a tea using basil leaves (using the basic tea recipe). Cool and strain for an effective insect bite or sting treatment.

Garlic Poultice

Crush a clove of garlic and apply it to the bite with an adhesive gauze bandage for twenty minutes. Do not leave it on too long, as garlic can actually burn the skin.

Lavender Oil

Place a drop of lavender oil on the sting or bite.

Marigold Tincture

This tincture (made according to the basic tincture recipe or purchased) also brings effective relief from gnat bites.

Ammonia Compress

Go no further than your housecleaning cupboard to find relief from insect bites. Simply dip a clean cloth in a few drops of ammonia diluted in one cup of water. Apply to bite. You can also do this with liquid laundry bluing.

Insect Bite Prevention

Taking thiamine (vitamin B1), 100 mg., three times a day, causes the body to secrete the vitamin. Most insects hate the odor, so they keep away!

Rubbing crushed pennyroyal leaves on your skin is another way to offend mosquitos and gnats. Ants hate goldenseal and black pepper, so sprinkle those herbs wherever the critters congregate.

Essential Oil Insect Repellent

Combine one tablespoon of any moisturizing cream with three drops of lavender oil and two drops of citronella oil. Add water for spreadable consistency and apply anywhere on your body, as needed. Either oil can be used separately. Geranium oil is also effective.

Garlic Insect Repellent

This might repel a few other creatures besides insects, but it works!

Simmer one cup of safflower or sunflower oil with one-half cup fresh feverfew blossoms or one tablespoon of the dried blossoms for twenty minutes. Remove from fire, cool slightly, and add eight well-chopped garlic cloves. Pour into a wide-mouthed jar or bottle and let the mixture stand for one week, shaking it a few times a day. Strain and apply to exposed skin, as needed. This also works as a remedy in case you forget to put it on before going out.

Insect Repellent Strips

Hang these easy-to-make strips in windows, open-air porches, or anywhere insects enter your home. Cut brown paper bags into one-half to one-inch strips. Place a drop of citronella oil at the bottom of each and hang.

Clothes Protector

Place a drop of marjoram oil in a small saucer and place it in your clothes closet to ward off moths and other insect invaders.

Mosquito Chaser

Make a strong decoction of chamomile flowers (using the basic tea recipe at two to three times normal strength). Use as a wash on exposed areas of the body to keep mosquitos away.

Cajeput Oil Repellent

This oil is used in Africa and India as a mosquito repellent. Apply to exposed areas of your body.

Feverfew Repellent

This infusion (made by doubling the amount of herbs in the basic tea recipe) will keep away gnats, mosquitos, and many other tiny winged critters. Simply sponge on this pleasant-smelling tea when it's cool, and let it dry.

Sweet Basil Repellent

Burn the dried leaves for a smoke that keeps mosquitos away.

Eucalyptus Repellent

Bruise the young leaves of eucalyptus and rub exposed areas of your body with them. You can also mix eucalyptus oil with glycerin and then apply to keep away mosquitos.

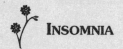 **INSOMNIA**

Milk is used as a natural sleep-inducer by many cultures all over the world. The reasons are calcium and tryptophan, an amino acid present in dairy products that is a proven promoter of REM-stage sleep, the most restful sleep period of the night. Many prescription sleep aids induce a drugged torpor that does not allow for REM sleep. You may sleep heavily, but you will not experience the benefits of a natural night's rest. However, if that REM stage is lengthened by natural means, the results are wonderfully beneficial to your overall health.

Soured Milk Products

Take a cup of either buttermilk, yogurt, or sour cream before bedtime.

Spanish-American Nightcap

Dissolve two tablespoons of honey in a glass of buttermilk. Stir in the juice of one lemon and mix well. The lemon ferments the milk, thus making it more digestible for those with lactose intolerance.

Catnip or Hops Tea

Brew one teaspoonful catnip or hops tea (using the basic tea recipe).

Chamomile Tea

Scientific studies have actually shown that a cup of chamomile tea (using the basic tea recipe) promotes a longer, deeper night's sleep.

Valerian-Skullcap-Catnip Tea

This soothing brew calms frazzled nerves and prepares you for a deep, relaxing sleep. Use equal parts of valerian, skullcap, and peppermint, totalling one teaspoon per one cup of boiling water. Steep for ten minutes.

Sour Tea

Drink either hot grapefruit or lemon juice, unsweetened.

Orange Ginseng Tea

Brew a decoction (using the basic decoction recipe) of equal parts orange peel and powdered ginseng root. Strain and add honey to taste. Drink just before bedtime to ensure a restful and revitalizing sleep.

Valerian Root

This helpful sleep aid can be combined with hops to make a mild sedative tea that promotes a healthy night's rest with no side effects. At bedtime, take one-half teaspoon of extract or 600 to 1000 mgs. in capsule form or brew one-half teaspoon of the dried herb to one cup of boiling water. Do not drink more than one cup a day.

Insomnia Combination Tea

Combine equal parts of chamomile, valerian, skullcap, catnip, wood betony, and spearmint. Use one ounce of herbs to one pint of boiling water. Steep for ten minutes. Drink before bedtime.

Knockout Tea

Do not drink more than one cup of this powerfully relaxing tea a day. In fact, it's best to space out mouthfuls so that you do not drink the tea all at once. Combine equal parts of valerian root, lady's slipper, skullcap, passionflower, and hops. Do not let the total amount of herbs used for one cup of tea exceed one-half teaspoon. (Passionflower is also effective when taken in tea form by itself.)

Primrose Tea

Primrose contains magnesium, which soothes frazzled nerves that can keep you sleepless. Brew according to the basic tea recipe and sip as needed before bedtime. If you mix it with milk, you add the sleep-inducing benefits of calcium.

Lettuce Tea

Simmer three or four chopped lettuce leaves in one and one-half cups of water for twenty minutes. Strain and drink before bedtime. Add a sprig of mint if a troubled stomach is keeping you awake.

Cider Vinegar

Soak a cotton pad in cider vinegar and then hold it under your nostrils as you lie in bed and inhale deeply. Lie still and sleep will soon overtake you.

Scottish Gruel

Cook oatmeal as usual but with more water so that the consistency is thin. Sweeten with honey to taste and drink at bedtime.

Raw Okra

They stock extra amounts of this vegetable in the South, where raw okra is a favored folk remedy known to induce sleepiness.

Coconut

Grind the meat of a coconut. Eat freely before bedtime to enjoy a peaceful night's rest.

Eye Compresses

A simple folk remedy for insomnia is to soak cotton pads in any warm solution, even plain water, and place them over the eyes. This relaxes you and prepares you for either sleep or a quick catnap.

Lavender Oil Soak

Fill a warm tub, then add ten to twenty drops of lavender oil and one cup of baking soda. Soak for twenty to thirty minutes. You'll feel relaxed, warm, and ready for a good night's rest.

Chamomile Relaxing Soak

Make a quart-sized decoction of chamomile flowers or linden flowers (following the basic tea recipe). Strain and add to your bath water. After you dry off, enjoy a cup of chamomile tea.

Sweet Dreams Pillow

Stuff a pillow case with hops. You can also stuff your pillow with equal parts hops and mugwort. Some people sprinkle their pillow with a little alcohol to bring out its soporific benefits. You can also place a cotton ball infused with one drop of lavender oil under your pillow to relax your nerves, relieve stress, and ensure a peaceful night's sleep.

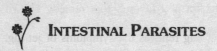

INTESTINAL PARASITES

See your doctor for an accurate diagnosis. Garlic, taken raw or three to six capsules a day, is a great parasite cure. In addition, try healing mild cases with the following remedies.

Garlic Worm Remedy

Peel two or three garlic cloves and mince well. Drop them into an eight-ounce glass and add warm water until the glass is about three-fourths full. Stir, cover, and allow to stand overnight. Strain in the morning and drink the water before you eat breakfast.

Amoebic Parasite Remedy

Simmer one teaspoon of mango bark in one cup of boiling water for at least ten minutes. Drink one cup, three times a day, until condition clears.

Papaya Leaf

If available, try eating one papaya leaf a day to rid your body of any parasite.

Pumpkin Seeds

Eat pumpkin seeds freely and use an herbal laxative to expel parasites and worms.

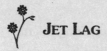

JET LAG

Ginseng

Siberian ginseng relieves the symptoms of jet lag. The Russians even gave the herb to their cosmonauts to help them adjust to the changes in biological rhythms they encountered in space. Take sixty drops (approximately one teaspoon) of extract (using the basic tincture recipe), three times a day, on an empty stomach. Or take one capsule, three or four times a day. For prevention, start taking the herb several days before leaving and for a couple of days following your flight.

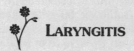

LARYNGITIS

Throat Soothing Tea

Pour one cup of boiling water over one teaspoon each of valerian root, skullcap, and catnip. Steep for ten to twenty minutes and sip while hot.

Laryngitis Steam

Boil water, remove from heat, and add the following essential oils: two drops of chamomile, three drops of lavender, two drops of thyme. Make a tent from a towel, lean over the pot, and inhale the steam until it dissipates.

Laryngitis Tea

Add one-quarter teaspoon of cayenne pepper and three to four drops of lemon juice to one cup of boiling water. Sip slowly while the liquid is hot.

Honey-Onion-Sugar Cough Syrup

This remedy is excellent for coughs, hoarseness, and whooping cough.

Peel and chop finely one pound of onions. Combine the onions with two ounces of honey, three-quarter pound of brown sugar, and two pints of water. Simmer over low heat for three hours. Cool, then bottle and cap well. Take four to six tablespoons spread out throughout the day.

Chamomile Sugar

This pep-up treat relieves coughs and hoarseness and provides a quick energy boost. Make chamomile oil by mxing one and one-half pints of safflower oil with three ounces of dried chamomile leaves. Simmer in a glass or stainless steel saucepan for forty minutes. Remove from heat and let stand overnight. Strain and bottle.

Combine the chamomile oil with equal parts date sugar, and take by the tablespoonful as needed.

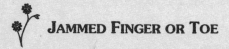

JAMMED FINGER OR TOE

Pour one tablespoon of olive oil over one or two large grated onions. Apply as a thick poultice to the injured finger or toe. Cover and secure well. The pain will disappear after a few minutes and any potential complications along with it.

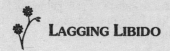

LAGGING LIBIDO

Licorice Water

Mix one teaspoon of powdered licorice root in a glass of plain soda. Drink as desired, to purify blood (and hence your complexion), nourish your glands, and invigorate your love life.

Bee Pollen

Studies have indicated that women who take courses of bee pollen tablets improve menopausal complaints, ease nervous conditions, and restore sexual function.

See your doctor before embarking on any bee pollen treatment as it can cause allergic reactions.

Damiana Tea

Damiana is a shrub found in desert areas of Mexico and Texas. It contains aromatic oils and other substances that stimulate the reproductive system and nervous system and boost circulation. More than just an aphrodisiac, damiana is used to strengthen the reproductive organs and as a tonic for the entire system.

Pour one cup of boiling water over one teaspoon of the dried leaves or one-quarter teaspoon of the powder. Take one tablespoon, three times a day.

Saw Palmetto Berries

These berries grow wild along the southern California coast and the southeast shore of the United States. They can be picked and eaten fresh for their overall tonic qualities, especially to the mucous membranes and the sex glands.

To use the dried berries for a tea, pour one-half pint of

boiling water on one ounce of saw palmetto. Steep until cool, strain, and bottle. Take one teaspoon, three times a day, or you can take the capsules according to bottle directions.

Damiana and Saw Palmetto Aphrodisiac Tea

Combine damiana with saw palmetto for a double tonic effect on the urinary and reproductive tracts and to ensure they do not become irritated. Use equal parts of each herb to make a basic tea. Or you can use the extract forms (using the basic tincture recipe). Mix one teaspoon of each per one cup of water. Drink one-half cup, three times a day.

Red Clover

A common plant found in meadows of North America and Europe, it is also known as purple clover. Red clover tea is calming, especially to those with infections. Substances in the blossoms are thought to have mild estrogenic effects that help prepare the body for lovemaking by stimulating lubrication. You can drink the tea (using the basic tea recipe) or take it in capsule form (follow bottle directions). But for aphrodisiac purposes, it's best to add two teaspoons of red clover extract (use the basic tincture recipe) to four ounces of red wine, as alcohol renders herbs more potent.

Ginseng Get-up

Several Indian tribes, and many Asian groups, used decoction of ginseng root as a sexual tonic, especially for males. Ginseng is not a powerful aphrodisiac, but its sustained energy-building effect works through the glands and normalizes many functions, including those that regulate sexual function. Taken as a tea, tincture, capsule, or even chewing on the root promotes an overall stimulating and energizing effect.

American Indian Ginseng Combination Tea

Mix together one tablespoon each of powdered ginseng root, parsley root, and wild columbine. Pour one and one-half pints of boiling water over the herb mixture. Cover and steep for ten to fifteen minutes. Strain. Drink one cup, three times a day, or as needed.

Fenugreek Seed Tea and Honey Treats

This valuable herb is rich in vitamin A, a lack of which is often found in men suffering from impotence. It also contains trimethylamine, which acts as a sex hormone in frogs and speeds up flower production in plants. Many cultures also use these seeds to cure male impotence and female sexual under-activity. You can drink the tea (using the basic decoction recipe) or try these tasty honey treats.

Grind the seeds into a powder. (Use a coffee grinder or a blender at high speed, or try an old-fashioned mortar and pestle.) Mix with an equal part of honey. Take by the table-spoonful as often as desired.

Sarsaparilla Root Extract

Sarsaparilla root contains sex-drive boosting hormones. Brew a tea (using the basic decoction recipe), or for more power, make a tincture (using the basic tincture recipe). Take a maximum of three cups a day of the tea or fifteen drops of the tincture, three times a day.

Sarsaparilla Sex Tonic

Bring two ounces of well-chopped sarsaparilla root to a boil in one quart of water. Cover and simmer for one-half hour. Cool, strain, and add a garnish of powdered ginger to each serving. Take one-half cup, three or four times a day, or as needed.

Pumpkin, Sesame, and Sunflower Seeds

Many ancient cultures have prized these seeds for their hormone-boosting qualities, especially for males. Sesame seeds mixed with honey are a centuries-old favorite for both sexes.

Sesame Combination Treat

This delicious dessert paste is a quick energy tonic and hormone booster. Simmer three tablespoons of sesame seed, one ounce of licorice root, and one-quarter pound of pitted, minced dates in two quarts of water until the liquid is reduced to one quart. Remove from heat and add one cup of honey, stirring well until the mixture is well blended. Take two tablespoons three or four times a day, or as needed.

Hops-Citrus Sex Tonic

Simmer the peel of two lemons and one orange in one quart of water for twenty minutes. Add three tablespoons of dried hops and simmer for three minutes. Remove from heat and stir in honey to taste. Cover and cool to lukewarm. Add three tablespoons of lecithin, mixing well. Take one-half cup, three or four times a day.

Gypsy Love Tea

Mix together one ounce each of hops, alfalfa, agrimony, and centaury. Add one quart of water and bring to a boil. Cover and simmer for fifteen minutes. Remove from heat, strain, and cool. Take one-half cup before meals, three times a day.

American Indian Libido Gruel

Bring two tablespoons of unrefined oatmeal, one-half cup of raisins, and one quart of water to a boil. Cover and simmer for forty-five minutes. Remove from heat and strain. Add honey to taste. Cool and add one-half teaspoon of lemon juice. Take one cup, as needed.

Fennel-Licorice Sex Tonic

Simmer two teaspoons of slightly crushed fennel seeds and one ounce of minced licorice root in one pint of water for twenty minutes. Let stand until cool. Strain. Take two tablespoons, twice a day.

LICE

Head Lice Remedy

Mix three to four drops of thyme oil in one tablespoon of shampoo. Apply to the scalp and hair and leave on for five minutes. Rinse thoroughly with warm water. To loosen the grip of the eggs, rinse again with equal parts vinegar and warm water, then cover the scalp with a shower cap for fifteen to twenty minutes. Comb out the hair with a fine-tooth comb designed to remove lice and their eggs. Repeat one week later if necessary.

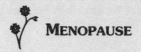

MENOPAUSE

Black Cohosh

Black cohosh balances the sex hormones and is the most widely used and effective treatment for the symptoms of menopause. Studies from Germany report that it relieves hot flashes, depression, anxiety, and vaginal atrophy associated with menopause without the side effects of hormones. Take one capsule, three times a day.

Dong Quai

This is another herb that balances the female system. Take one capsule, three times a day.

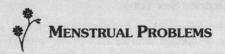

MENSTRUAL PROBLEMS

Many herbs nourish and tone the glandular system that controls female reproduction and the menstrual cycle, as well as related organ systems.

Amenorrhea Cure

Chaste berry extract is an effective restorative of the monthly cycle when bleeding has ceased. This herb can restore normal ovulation and bleeding by changing the release of hormones by the pituitary (prolactin, LH, FSH). When this happens, more progesterone is released, which also relieves premenstrual syndrome. The normal dosage is 175 to 225 mg. daily.

Female Regulator

Dong quai is also helpful in a variety of female complaints, including menopause symptoms such as hot flashes, and any abnormal menstrual pattern. It is best taken in capsules or extract.

Licorice Root

Like dong quai, licorice is an estrogen/progesterone precursor. If excess estrogen is causing the cramps, either herb fills up the binding sites, so the excess estrogen can be eliminated. If the problem is insufficient estrogen, either herb will provide stimulation. Take one capsule, three times a day. Licorice root can also be taken as a tea (using the basic tea recipe). Its gentle, supportive action make it suitable for long-term use.

Black Cohosh Tonic

Like licorice root, black cohosh is a nourishing tonic for the female system, particularly the uterus, due to the action of the phytoestrogens, which have estrogenic effects. It can be taken in capsule or tincture form.

Raspberry Leaf Tea

Pour one cup of boiling water over one teaspoon of raspberry leaves, which contain high levels of absorbable calcium. Steep for five minutes. Drink one cup, three times a day, to relieve painful menstruation. Some holistic healers report that raspberry leaf tea is effective during pregnancy but not for the relief of menstrual cramps.

Raspberry Cooler

Combine one ounce red raspberry leaves with one ounce red clover and place in a quart canning jar. Pour one quart boiling water over the herbs. Steep for three to four hours, then add cold water. Use lime juice to flavor.

Raspberry-Motherwort Tea

These herb teas can be taken together or separately. Pour two cups of boiling water over two teaspoons of the leaves. Brew for five minutes and drink as often and as much as desired.

Cramp Relieving Tea

Combine one tablespoon each of angelica root, cramp bark, and chamomile with one teaspoon of ginger root. Brew a tea (using the basic decoction recipe). Take one-half cup, three times a day.

Cramp Poultice

Make a poultice by mixing water with catnip powder or well-chopped leaves. Apply to lower abdomen and leave on until relief is obtained.

Tropical Menstrual Flow Reducer

Eat a mixture made of equal parts guava fruit and ground coconuts to prevent excessive menstrual flow.

Castor Oil Packs

An old-fashioned but highly effective treatment is to apply castor oil directly to the lower abdomen, cover with flannel or cheesecloth and a hot water bottle.

Valerian Root

Take one-half teaspoon of the tincture, followed by another one-half teaspoon, twenty minutes to one-half hour later.

Cramp Bark

Either take one capsule, three times daily or drink the tea, one cup, three times daily or more often, if necesary. This herb provides effective relief against strong cramps.

Gentle Cramp Relief

If the cramps are less severe, you can take tea made from either ginger, peppermint, or chamomile.

Juniper Berry Tea

Use juniper berries to make a tea (using the basic tea recipe) that relieves menstrual and other cramps. *Do not use if you are pregnant as this tea is a powerful relaxant and can induce labor*. Some traditional herbalists give this tea to women *after* labor has already started.

Endometriosis Relief

Many healers feel this condition is caused by dietary fat, particularly the fat found in dairy foods. So a change in diet is highly recommended. Other recommendations include flaxseed oil, two to three tablespoons a day; hot castor oil compresses three evenings per week, and three times a day doses of chaste or hemp tree (*Vitex agnus castus*), taken in extract, capsule, or syrup form. Dong quai can be used as a tea or taken in capsules, along with raspberry leaf and nettles.

PMS Eliminator

Oil of evening primrose helps reduce breast soreness and menstrual mood swings. Take six to nine 500 mg. capsules daily, preferably on a full stomach. It should start working by the third month.

For Uterine Inflammation

Combine one ounce each of the following: motherwort, skullcap, water betony, water dock, black horehound. Boil in five pints of water for thirty minutes. Towards the end, add one-half teaspoon of ginger. Strain. Take one-half cup, four times a day, before meals.

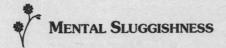

MENTAL SLUGGISHNESS

Rosemary Wine

Chop up one cup of green rosemary sprigs. Place in one pint of white wine. Strain off after a few days. Sip to stimulate the brain and nervous system.

Rosemary Tea

This tea (made according to the basic tea recipe) is said to stimulate the brain and sharpen your mental powers.

Gingko Biloba

Take two capsules, three or four times a day, to improve short-term memory. You can also take the tincture.

Hazelnuts

Eat hazelnuts daily.

Memory-Enhancing Teas

Brew teas (using the basic tea recipe) from any of the following herbs: chickweed, sweet flag, marigold, or licorice root.

Amish Pepper Seed Remedy

Eat green pepper seeds for nine days, beginning with one seed and doubling the dose until you reach 256 seeds on the ninth day. You know it's working if you can do this.

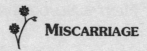

MISCARRIAGE

Red Raspberry Tea

Some herbalists report amazing results on women prone to miscarriages with this herb. Drink three to four cups of red raspberry tea (using the basic tea recipe) every day during pregnancy. Red raspberry is said to strengthen the attachment of the fetus to the uterus and even ease delivery at birth.

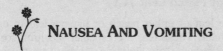 **NAUSEA AND VOMITING**

Antinausea Tea

Add two teaspoons of gentian root tincture and one teaspoon of peppermint tincture to two cups boiling water. Simmer for twenty minutes. Take one-half cup at a time, as needed.

Vinegar Drink

Mix one teaspoon of apple cider vinegar in one cup of water. Sip slowly. This works if your stomach lacks sufficient acidity.

Stomach Settling Tea

Mix together three tablespoons of cinnamon powder with one tablespoon each of powdered cardamom, nutmeg, and cloves. Steep one-half teaspoon of the herb mixture in one cup of hot water for ten minutes. Strain. Add honey to taste. Drink one cup as needed.

Peppermint Oil Drink

Mix one drop of peppermint oil in one-half cup of water. Sip slowly.

Morning Sickness Tea

Raspberry leaf tea (using the basic tea recipe) is recommended by herbalists to combat morning sickness. It is also beneficial to drink at least one cup a day throughout pregnancy.

Papaya or Peach Leaf Tea

Steep one leaf of either peach or papaya leaf in one cup of boiling water. These teas are especially helpful for pregnant women suffering from morning sickness or those who are chronically nauseous.

Motion Sickness Cure

Ginger root capsules have been found to be more effective than Dramamine in preventing the nausea of motion sickness. Take one or two capsules every three hours. You can also chew on the ginger stick or drink ginger tea. Or you can suck on a lemon wedge or chew several whole cloves, until the motion sickness passes.

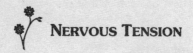

NERVOUS TENSION

Instead of popping prescription tranquilizers that dull rather than calm your nerves and cause harmful side effects, munch on either soybeans, rice polishings, bran, or carob candies— all of which soothe the nerves by nutritional means. The following are other healthful ways you can "mellow out."

Summer Calmer

This delicious drink is wonderfully cooling and calms nerves. Combine one-half ounce chamomile and one-half ounce lemon balm with enough pure water to make one quart. Place herbs in a quart canning jar and pour one quart boiling water over them. Close the lid tightly and allow the mixture to steep for three to four hours at room temperature. Dilute with cold water, and add honey and lemon to taste.

Dandelion Root Tea

If you're still drinking coffee or caffeinated teas, try dandelion root tea instead. It actually calms nerves and induces sleep. Roast dandelion roots until they are brown and hard. Grind them into a powder and store in a tightly capped jar. Brew as you would ordinary coffee, and drink freely, as desired. You can also purchase dandelion "coffee" at a health food store.

Valerian Root

Valerian root, in capsule or extract form, has a powerfully relaxing effect on the parasympathetic nervous system. It is also useful in treating headaches. If you are also suffering from a headache and upset stomach, brew a tea, combining valerian with peppermint. While valerian is an excellent sedative, it is also allergenic for some people. Try a small amount the first time you use it.

Sage Balancer

Sage has been found to have an action on the cortex of the brain which is beneficial to nervous tension, mental exhaustion, strengthens powers of concentration, and promotes relaxation. Use the basic tea recipe.

Lady's Slipper Tea

This herb is usually taken in tincture form, but for a mild, safe, soothing drink that calms jangled nerves, brew a tea from the roots, steeping one ounce in one quart of boiling water for twenty to thirty minutes. Take one cup every hour or two until symptoms subside.

Nerve-Soothing Combination Tea

Combine equal parts of the following herb powders: lady's slipper, valerian, wood betony, skullcap, spearmint, lemon balm. Mix well and steep two tablespoons of the herbal mixture in one cup of hot water for ten minutes. Add honey to taste. Drink as needed, up to three cups a day.

Celery Combination Nerve Tea

Simmer one-third cup of fresh, chopped celery stalks and leaves in two and one-half cups of boiling water for fifteen minutes. Strain. Place one heaping teaspoon each of chamomile and hops in a pot. Reheat the celery water to boiling and pour over the herb mixture. Cover and steep for five minutes. Take one-half to one cup twice a day, or as needed.

Celery Tea

While not recommended if you have acute kidney problems or are pregnant, celery tea, made from the seeds and stalks as in the above remedy, is excellent for nervousness. (Only six drops of the oil extracted from the root is said to restore potency impaired by illness.)

Catnip Tea

Pour one cup of boiling water over one teaspoon of catnip leaves. Steep for five minutes.

Vervain Leaf

Taken in capsules, one, three times a day, this plant calms nerves. It is also a general tonic and cleanser, and makes an effective lotion for the eyes.

Lavender Whiff

A whiff of the oil acts on the brain's limbic system, which controls the nervous system and protects the brain from overstimulation. Calm your nerves with just a drop of lavender oil placed on a finger and sniffed.

Lemon Balm Stress Eliminator

Lemon balm is often used in essential oil form. The oil contains citronellol, which can cause a slight skin irritation in some people. Add twenty drops of oil to bath water.

Sleep-inducing Soak

Thyme is another popular ingredient in herb pillows that calms nerves. Steep a few handfuls in one gallon of cold water for twelve hours. Heat slowly to a gentle boil, then simmer for ten minutes. Strain, then add the strained liquid to your bath water. If you have sensitive skin, use the dried herb. The essential oil may cause rashes.

Valerian Bath

Valerian has a soothing and tonifying affect on the nervous system even when used externally. To prepare a valerian bath, boil one pound of the herb in a large pot of water. Boil for thirty minutes. Strain and add to bath water.

Goldenrod Soothing Soak

This herb is taken from a flower common to North America. Even if you're normally allergic to goldenrod, you probably can use it in a soak because once it's dried, most of the pollen is gone.

Lavender Bath

Lavender flowers make for a calming bath that is also said to relieve pains of rheumatism and gout. Pour one pound of the herb in a large pot of boiling water. Cover, remove from heat, and allow to stand for fifteen minutes. Add to bath water.

Hops/Meadowsweet Rinse

Make a warm decoction of equal parts hops and meadow-sweet (using the basic tea recipe). Pour over your entire body after your regular bath or shower.

Pine Oil Bath

Add one tablespoon of pine oil to your bath water. This bath relieves tension and strain while it stimulates the circulation and refreshes your system.

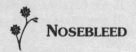

NOSEBLEED

A few drops of onion juice placed in the nose while the head is held back will arrest a nosebleed.

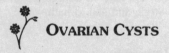

OVARIAN CYSTS

Warning: Be sure that your doctor monitors your progress, as a ruptured cyst can be life-threatening.

Herbal Cyst Program

Combine one ounce each of raspberry leaves, black currant leaves, witch hazel leaves, and powdered myrrh. Boil in one quart of water in a covered pot for ten minutes, then simmer for one-half hour. Strain. Mix one-half cup of this mixture with one pint of distilled water. Use this liquid as a nightly douche. Make sure your bowels are moving properly.

In addition, combine one ounce each of dandelion, comfrey, yellow dock, and yarrow with two ounces of licorice root. Divide the mixture into three parts. Add one pint of boiling distilled water to each third, as you use it. Simmer for twenty minutes. Cool and strain. Take one tablespoon, three times a day.

For Ovary Inflammation

Combine one ounce each of motherwort, water dock, black horehound, and sunflower. Simmer in five pints of distilled water for thirty minutes. Strain. Take one-half cup four times a day. This reduces inflammation and tones the ovaries.

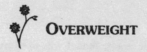 **OVERWEIGHT**

Diets do not work. The only effective way to take off weight and keep it off is to practice good nutrition throughout your life, avoiding sugars, refined carbohydrates, excessive fats, and eating whole foods. Regular exercise is essential. The following remedies will help.

Herbal Diuretics

If you do not take caffeine regularly and your body hasn't built up a tolerance, ordinary tea will work as a diuretic, ridding your body temporarily of excess fluids. Healthier alternatives include steeping one teaspoon of either dried cornsilk, horsetail (which also stimulates metabolism), uva ursi, or parsley seed in one cup of boiling water for five minutes. Drink one cup, three times a day.

Hawthorn

An even stronger diuretic, hawthorn is best taken by capsule or tincture. Take two capsules or one dropperful of the tincture, three times a day.

Dandelion Leaves

Dandelion leaves work especially well as a diuretic, plus the leaves contain five percent potassium, which can be depleted by synthetic diuretics.

Milk Thistle

Milk thistle is particularly effective during the holidays. It reduces bloating, aids in digestion of sweets, and helps protect the liver against overindulgence in alcohol.

Fennel Tea

During the Middle Ages, fennel was used by Christians during fasting periods to stave away hunger pains. It is also a diuretic and highly recommended for weight loss.

Herbal Appetite Control Capsules

Mix together equal parts of the following herbal powders: saffron, burdock, parsley, kelp, licorice, fennel, echinacea, black walnut, papaya, hawthorn berries, and mandrake. Fill 00-size gelatin capsules. Take two capsules before each meal together with two capsules of chickweed.

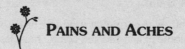

PAINS AND ACHES

Mustard Plasters

Surprisingly, the old-fashioned mustard plaster is still an excellent treatment for sore, stiff muscles or a sore back. It draws blood to the area which helps to loosen the muscles and carry away toxins that cause the muscles to tighten and spasm.

Mix mustard seed powder with enough distilled water to make a paste. Apply to the affected area and cover.

Linseed Poultice

Like mustard plasters, this oil makes a good poultice for spastic muscles. It is also effective for softening boils.

Allspice (Pimento)

Allspice, grown in Jamaica, makes an excellent stimulating plaster for the relief of rheumatism and neuralgia. Boil fresh berries in water until the mixture is thick enough to be spread on linen or cheesecloth. Apply to affected area. (Pimento oil, made from the green leaves of the plant, is useful for flatulence and indigestion.)

Nettles Treat

A plant commonly found along roadsides and in meadows, nettle eases sprains, joint and muscle pain, and inflammation with its refreshing and energizing effects.

Soak eight ounce of dried nettles in one gallon of cold water for twelve hours. Heat, strain, and add to footbath. Or bruise the leaves and make a poultice for the affected area.

Herbal Soak Balm

This herbal bath is the formula used in Europe's most exclusive spas to soothe exhausted and aching muscles. Steep equal parts of dried thyme, field horsetail, goldenrod, and lemon balm. You should wind up with approximately three ounces or a few handfuls in total. Steep in one gallon of cold water for twelve hours. Heat slowly to a gentle boil. Strain the herbs and add the liquid to your bath water. Since some of the herbs may not be beneficial to your heart, be sure that the water is just deep enough to cover your lower back.

Painful Joint Poultice

Combine the following herb powders:

> 3 parts plantain
> 3 parts comfrey
> 1 part marshmallow root
> 1 part lobelia
> ⅛ part cayenne

Mix together well. Add equal parts of either honey, wheat germ oil, olive oil, or vitamin E oil to make a paste. Cover with bandage and secure well. Leave on for twenty-four hours. (This also works well to draw out infections.)

Garlic Ointment

This pungent ointment provides a soothing deep heat when rubbed into aching and stiff joints. It also works well as a chest rub for colds, lung congestion, and bronchitis.

Place three-quarters cup of minced garlic and one cup of pure lard in a jar. Set the jar in a pan of boiling water. Stir occasionally for three hours as the lard melts, replacing the hot water as needed. Remove from heat and let cool until the mixture solidifies. Stir well and cover tightly. Use as a rub when needed.

Herbal Liniment

Combine one ounce of powdered myrrh, one-half ounce of powdered goldenseal, one-quarter ounce of cayenne pepper, and one pint rubbing alcohol. Mix together and let stand for seven days, shaking a few times every day. Then pour the liquid into another bottle, leaving the sediment behind.

Rub sore, aching areas for fifteen to twenty minutes, three to four times a day. If you can't rub directly over the sore spot, rub the surrounding area.

Tiger Balm

A popular remedy from China, tiger balm is made from oil of camphor in a petroleum base. After rubbing the sore, aching area, in approximately ten minutes, you will feel intense heat on that spot. It's also excellent for breaking up the congestion of a cold.

Onion Poultice

Finely chop one onion and mix with two tablespoons of honey or sugar. Spread on a cloth and apply to the sprain.

Horseradish Poultice

Fresh chopped or grated horseradish mixed with a little water makes an effective pain-reliever and circulation booster for rheumatism and stiffness and pain, particularly in the neck area. You can also make a heat-delivering compress by boiling the horseradish in milk for fifteen to twenty minutes.

Circulation Boosting Poultice

Combine one tablespoon of powdered ginger root and cayenne with one-half tablespoon of powdered lobelia and enough olive oil to make a paste. Apply to affected areas, bandage, and secure well.

Amish Tennis Elbow Rub

Add four freshly chopped avocado seeds and three ounces of horsetail grass to one quart of water. Bring to a boil and cook down to one pint. Add one pint of rubbing alcohol. Rub as needed into sore area.

Back Pain Rub

Boil two tablespoons of cayenne pepper in one pint of cider vinegar for ten minutes. Cool and apply while still warm. Use for any sore area.

Rosemary Oil Rub

Soak the plant's tops and leaves in a pure, cold-pressed vegetable oil for one week. Use as a rub on sore or sprained areas.

Comfrey Poultice

Fresh leaves are best, but if you can't get them, you can use the dried leaves or the chopped roots. Place a generous handful in a pan, cover with water and bring to a boil. Remove the pan from the heat if you are using the leaves. If you are using the roots, maintain a slow, rolling boil for twenty to thirty minutes. Let the mixture cool to the point where it's warm. Place on affected area between layers of gauze. If your skin becomes irritated, coat it with olive oil before applying the poultice. This poultice is especially effective for bursitis.

Balkan Bone and Joint Pain Remedy

This remedy came to this country from the country villages of the Balkans. It requires a bottle which holds nine-tenths of a quart. Fill the bottle three-fourths full with vodka and the balance with the flowers and small tops of rosemary. Tightly seal the bottle and place in the hot sun for three days. If the sun is not hot enough or there is no sun, keep the bottle near a heated stove or on the pilot light. Shake the mixture well three times a day. After three days, strain the liquid carefully and place in another bottle with two or three grains of camphor. Shake well as soon as the camphor dissolves. Rub small amounts of the mixture into the skin over the affected areas until the skin will absorb no more. Stop rubbing and cover the affected areas with wool or flannel.

Flaxseed Poultices

As you pour one pint of boiling water into a warmed enamel or glass pan, simultaneously sprinkle in one-quarter pound of crushed flaxseeds. Stir until the mixture has the consistency of a smooth dough. Add one-half ounce of olive oil. Spread the mixture on a clean cloth. Fold it over and apply to affected area. You can also use less flaxseed and add some slippery elm and marshmallow powder. This poultice is also very helpful for bursitis.

Pain-Easing Tea

Combine two tablespoons of chamomile with one tablespoon of powdered skullcap and one tablespoon of roughly ground root of lady's slipper. If you are taking this tea at bedtime, add one tablespoon each of hops and passion flower. Using the basic decoction recipe, bring to boil and simmer for fifteen to twenty minutes. Strain and sip.

Willow Bark Tea

Willow bark is the main ingredient in aspirin and other commercial pain relievers. Soak one-half teaspoon of powdered willow bark in two cups of water overnight. Bring the mixture to a boil, then simmer for twenty to thirty minutes. Strain and cool. Keep in refrigerator and use when needed. Take only one-quarter cup at a time and sip slowly.

Oil of Cajeput Massage

This oil has a deep, penetrating action. Apply directly, gently massaging and manipulating the sore and aching muscles.

American Indian Sunflower–Witch Hazel Liniment

This liniment is also effective on sore muscles and sprains. Mix together equal parts of distilled witch hazel and sunflower seed oil.

Camphorated Olive Oil

Another great remedy for sore muscles and sprains is made by mixing together equal parts of camphor and olive oil and rubbing on affected areas.

Chamomile Oil

To prepare the oil, place three ounces of chamomile leaves in one and one-half pints of pure, cold-pressed vegetable oil. Simmer in a glass or stainless steel saucepan for forty minutes. Remove from heat and let stand overnight. Strain and bottle. Rub into painful joints as frequently as desired.

Combination Liniment

Combine one ounce each of sunflower seed oil, turpentine oil, camphor oil, clove oil, and wintergreen oil. This powerful liniment works on sprains, sore muscles, and helps alleviate the pain of rheumatism and arthritis.

Combination Liniment II

Dissolve one-third teaspoon of dry camphor and one-third teaspoon of dry mustard seed in one pint of turpentine. Add one pint of any pure, cold-pressed vegetable oil and one pint of rubbing alcohol. Allow to steep for a few days, shaking a few times a day. Shake well each time you use it. Massage into painful areas, allowing the skin to absorb as much liniment as possible. Apply a flannel wrapping to cover. This is equally effective in relieving chest congestion.

Rosemary Oil

Boil one handful of rosemary leaves in one pint of pure, cold-pressed vegetable oil for twenty minutes. Cool, strain, and bottle with tight-fitting cap.

Make a hot compress of either sour milk or buttermilk and apply to sore and strained muscles.

Lard Ointment

This may be unappetizing, but it's effective! Simmer one cup of marigold flowers and leaves in one cup of lard for twenty minutes. Strain, cool, and bottle.

Iron-out Pain Cure

Moisten a flannel cloth with vinegar. Place the cloth over the sore area. Glide a hot iron over the cloth as if you were ironing a piece of clothing. Keep doing this until relief is obtained.

Vinegar Cast

Cut a brown paper bag into strips one inch wide. Dip the strips in vinegar. One by one, wrap the strips around the affected joint or area and let them dry to form a homemade "cast" that supports the painful area and provides soothing relief.

Muscular Ache and Pain Baths

Baths prepared with balm and other "hot" and "sweet" herbs have been used since antiquity to ease weary and aching muscles. Mugwort was added to bathwater by the Romans to ease the vigors of war. For best results, stay in the bath for twenty minutes or more, massaging aching muscles.

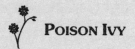 **POISON IVY**

Plaintain Leaves

Crush the leaves of this common weed and rub on affected area for dramatic relief of itching.

Baking Soda

Either a baking soda solution or poultice is very soothing and promotes healing.

Aloe Vera Gel

The juice from this succulent's leaves is healing to burns as well as poison ivy blisters.

Brown Soap, Calamine Lotion, Vitamin E

Apply brown soap to the affected areas and allow it to dry. Or you can apply calamine lotion or vitamin E oil, particularly to areas that you have scratched raw.

Comfrey Poultices

Comfrey is extremely effective in healing all manner of skin disorders, from poison ivy to superficial infections. Use according to the basic poultice recipe. To prevent possible skin irritation, coat the affected area with olive oil or lanolin before applying the poultice.

American Indian Poison Ivy and Oak Cure

Mash the fresh stems and leaves of impatiens, also known as jewel weed. Pour off the juice and apply to the affected areas. This remedy is not only an effective treatment, it can be used as a preventive. Simply rub the fresh juice on exposed areas of skin before going into any areas where poison ivy or poison oak may be growing.

Garlic Poultice

Crush several garlic cloves and place between layers of gauze. Apply to the affected areas for one-half hour.

Combination Poultice

This works well for either poison oak or poison ivy.

Combine equal parts of macerated comfrey root, marshmallow root, slippery elm, aloe vera, and witch hazel leaves. Apply to affected areas, cover, and secure.

Combination Poultice II

Combine equal parts of macerated mugwort, plantain, and comfrey leaves. Apply to affected areas, cover, and secure.

Poison Oak and Poison Ivy Tea

Purify your blood as part of the cure, using this powerfully cleansing tea.

Combine the following herb powders:

> 1 tablespoon chaparral
> 2 tablespoons yellow dock
> 2 tablespoons echinacea

Make a tea (using the basic tea recipe). Take one cup every two hours, until itching subsides.

Cider Vinegar Solution

Mix cider vinegar with an equal part of water. Sponge on affected areas twice daily and allow to dry.

Alum and Vaseline

Mix together powdered alum with enough Vaseline to make a paste. Apply to affected areas.

Lobelia Wash

Make a strong tea, doubling the amount of lobelia in the basic tea recipe. Cool and strain. Apply to affected area.

Fruit Rub

Rub the inside of the skin of banana, orange, or lemon on the affected areas.

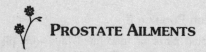

PROSTATE AILMENTS

Between forty to fifty percent of men past the age of fifty-five experience benign prostatic hyperplasia (BPH), commonly known as an enlarged prostate. Inflammation or enlargement of the prostate is far more common than active infections or progressive diseases. But if left untreated, an enlarged or irritated prostate can lead to bladder infections, kidney damage, and impotence. A diet high in fats is generally considered to be a contributing factor, and many men have cured or prevented BPH by using natural remedies. You must, however, consult your doctor before beginning any regimen, particularly since the symptoms for prostatic cancer and enlarged prostate are similar.

Saw Palmetto

Extract of saw palmetto berry has been found to normalize prostate function. It decreases the frequency of urination, relieves difficulty in urination, and lessens the inflammation and pain associated with BPH. This remedy has a long history of use with Amerian Indian groups. Take 160 mg. of a standardized (85–90 percent) extract, twice daily.

Healthy Prostate Tea

Brew a tea (using the basic tea recipe) from equal parts of buchu leaves, uva ursi, and saw palmetto. This is a particularly helpful drink following a prostate operation to soothe irritation and speed healing.

Burdock Tea

Brew a tea from the roots, using the basic decoction recipe. Take one cup, three times a day.

Prostate Tonic

This formula is said to dissolve kidney stones and cure prostate infections.

Combine one-half ounce each of powdered gravel root, uva ursi, parsley root, goldenseal root, cayenne, juniper berries, and marshmallow root with one-quarter ounce of powdered licorice root.

Mix together well and fill 00-size gelatin capsules. Take two capsules, twice a day, with one-half cup of warm water, at least one-half hour before meals.

Prostate Tonic II

This decoction is effective in cases of inflammation.

Combine one-half ounce each of powdered gravel root, uva ursi, echinacea, and parsley root with one-eighth ounce each of powdered ginger root and lobelia. Make a tea (using the basic decoction recipe). Strain. Drink three to four cups a day until relief is obtained.

Ginseng

Studies report that panax ginseng increases testosterone levels and decreases the size of the prostate. The suggested dose is 2 to 4 grams of the dried root in capsule form, taken three times a day. Or you can take an extract standardized to 17 percent ginsenosides (the active ingredients in ginseng).

Bee Pollen

Europeans have used bee pollen to treat BPH since the early 1960's. Bee pollen is also an excellent antibacterial for prostate infections. Take two teaspoons of raw bee pollen each day.

Pumpkin Seeds

Baked and pulverized pumpkin seeds are a popular remedy for prostate problems because they contain the building elements for male hormones. (These seeds are also a great preventative and remedy for worm infestation.) Chronic prostate infections are linked to a lack of dietary zinc. Pumpkin seeds are a rich source of zinc, as well as essential fatty acids, which are also necessary for prostate health.

Pumpkin Seed Prostate Tonic

Simmer four ounces of whole pumpkin seeds in one quart of water for twenty minutes. Cool and pour into a wide-mouth bottle. Cool and allow the seeds to settle at the bottom. Stir well each time you use. Take one-half cup, three times a day or as needed.

If chlamydia, the most common cause of nonbacterial prostatitis, is the culprit, take one-half to one teaspoon of goldenseal root extract three times daily or one 250- to 500-mg. goldenseal capsule three times a day. You can also take 500 to 1000 mg. of the freeze-dried leaves three times daily or one-quarter to one-half teaspoon of the fluid extract, three times a day.

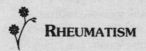 # RHEUMATISM

In cases of both arthritis and rheumatism, it's best to avoid the nightshade plants such as tomatoes, eggplant, green peppers, and potatoes, as well as sugar, pork, and strawberries.

Celery Milk

Celery cooked in milk is a great rheumatism remedy. It neutralizes uric acid and other excess acids, and its alkaline reaction in the body relieves rheumatism. Celery also contains valuable minerals, particularly sodium. Organic sodium keeps inorganic calcium in solution until it can be eliminated, thus helping to prevent and cure arthritis. Do not use if you have serious kidney problems.

Celery Water

Chop up a bunch of celery and boil until soft in two quarts of water. Drink as much as you want, three or four times a day.

At the same time, place the cooked celery in a pot with two pints of milk. Add a little flour to thicken and a few dashes of nutmeg. Serve warm with toast.

Another option is to use celery extract, decoction, or powder.

Grape Root Blood Purifier

The first step in healing many ailments is often an effective blood purifier. This one is particularly good for rheumatism and arthritis.

Mix together the following herbs:

> 6 tablespoons oregon grape root
> 6 tablespoons parsley root
> 3 tablespoons sassafras
> 3 tablespoons prickly ash bark
> 3 tablespoons black cohosh
> 3 tablespoons guaiacum
> 2 tablespoons ginger root

Chop the herbs finely. Make a tea (using the basic decoction recipe). Simmer for thirty minutes. Take one-half cup every two hours.

Cornsilk Tea

Valued also for its soothing effect on irritated bladders, this tea made from the silky hairs that line corn husks is also a good liver tonic, especially for those suffering from rheumatism. Boil one and one-half tablespoons of corn silk in one and one-half cups of water for ten minutes. Strain and drink hot, as needed. Sweeten with honey to taste.

Devil's Claw

Taken either in tea, pill, extract, or capsule form, this herb from Latin America is said to relieve arthritis and rheumatism. Take according to the package directions.

Aloe Vera Juice

Drink three ounces of the pure juice, three times a day.

Amish Tea

Combine one-half ounce each of burdock, yellow dock root, sassafras bark, dandelion, and dwarf elder. Boil in two quarts of water until the liquid reduces to one quart. Take two table-spoons, three times a day, at least one-half hour before meals.

Rheumatism Soother

Boil one cup of bran in one quart of water. Soak painful parts in the water for fifteen minutes. Then apply onion layers over the area and bind with a cloth. At midnight, rise and remove the onions and bathe the affected part with water. Put the onion poultice in place again until morning. Repeat until results are obtained.

Rheumatism and Arthritis Stiff Joint Remedy

Place two pounds of fresh birch leaves (or one pound dried) in an old pillowcase. Boil gently in two gallons of water for forty minutes. Add both the bag and the water to your bath and soak for at least half an hour. If you don't live near birch trees, try pine needles if they're available.

Honeysuckle

One tasty way to consume this flower is a handful of fresh blossoms with a few leaves. If that is not possible, brew a tea from the dried flowers and leaves (using the basic tea recipe). Take one cup, three times a day.

Plums

Plums, known for their laxative effect, are also an effective remedy for rheumatism. Either eat the fruit whole or brew a tea, using a handful of plums to one quart of water. Simmer for twenty minutes. Strain off the plums (and eat them separately), and drink the remaining plum tea freely.

Dandelion Tea

Brew a tea from the fresh leaves, if possible (using the basic tea recipe). Drink one cup, three or four times a day.

Nettle Tea

Brew a strong tea from nettles (using the basic decoction recipe). Take one cup, three times a day to help heal rheumatism.

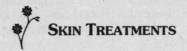

SKIN TREATMENTS

Comfrey Ointment

Mix three parts of comfrey leaves or roots with one-half part of honey and one and one-half parts of wheat germ oil or Vitamin E oil. This healing ointment is effective for minor burns, skin ulcers, sprains, fractures, and cuts. The vitamin E and honey soothe the skin and also promote healing.

Combination Healing Oinment

Combine two ounces of calendula flowers with one ounce each of crushed plantain leaves, mugwort, and crushed comfrey leaves.

Macerate the herbs and saute four ounces of the mixture in one pint of olive oil over a low heat until the herbs are crisp. Strain out the herbs and store. This ointment is useful for skin rashes, swellings, wounds, cuts, and burns.

Powdered Goldenseal Poultices

Also effective, even for skin lesions. (Use the basic poultice recipe.)

Red Clover Rash Poultice

Make a strong red clover tea and let it steep for thirty to forty minutes. Apply to the rash and let it dry. Repeat frequently. It is helpful to also take the tea internally at the same time.

Eczema Poultice

Brew a decoction made of equal parts of comfrey root, witch hazel bark, and white oak bark, with one-half teaspoon of goldenseal. Soak a clean cloth in the decoction and apply to the affected area. If the condition is on the feet or hands, a simple soak is easier and just as effective. This treatment and the one that follows are for symptoms only. Both eczema and psoriasis are indicative of an underlying medical condition that must be diagnosed and treated.

Eczema Soother

Mix together well equal parts of zinc oxide ointment and lanolin. (You can buy both at your local drugstore.) Add an equal amount of garlic powder (available at supermarkets and health food stores), a little at a time to prevent lumping. Or blend at low speed in your blender. When the mixture is thoroughly blended, store in tightly covered jar. Use as needed.

Papaya Poultice

The juice from this delicious fruit, either applied directly or with a clean cloth or piece of gauze, is also an excellent remedy for acne and freckles and it helps remove dead skin, leaving your skin baby-soft and smooth.

Horseradish Milk Freckle Solution

This freckle fading remedy comes from the Gypsies. Simmer one cup of grated or scraped horseradish in one pint of boiled milk for fifteen to twenty minutes. Cool and apply to skin.

Leave it to dry for half an hour, then wash off with tepid water. Repeat every two or three days, until the freckles fade away.

Mango Skin Smoother

Grind the fruit of mangoes into a pulp. Rub it all over your body to tone the skin and unclog pores.

Psoriasis Soother

Brew a strong decoction made of equal parts comfrey root and goldenseal. Soak a clean cloth in the decoction and apply to the affected area.

Natural Antibacterial Paste

This remedy works very well on impetigo, a highly contagious infection that often appears around the mouth. Mix echinacea and goldenseal powder with a little pure water until they form a paste. Spread over the affected skin with gauze or cotton. Cover well and secure to prevent spreading the infection.

Oatmeal Bath

Aveeno oatmeal, mixed in bath water, is recommended even by dermatologists to relieve itchy skin and contact dermatitis. Or you can use any good quality oatmeal.

Another way to take an oatmeal bath is to fill a cloth bag with one pound of oatmeal. Tie securely and place in the warm bathwater. Stay in the tub for twenty minutes at least, rubbing the skin with the oatmeal bag.

Borage Skin Rash Poultice

This remedy is effective against many types of rashes, including ringworm. Place one cup of fresh borage leaves in a blender with two or three tablespoons of water. Blend to a thick pulp. Spread the pulp on a piece of clean cloth or gauze and then apply to the rash, taping securely. Leave on overnight. Repeat until the rash is gone.

Tea Tree Oil

This essential oil is distilled from the leaves of the tree that grows on the north coast of New South Wales, Australia, and imported heavily to North America and elsewhere. Apply the oil directly to fungal skin infections. Tea tree also makes a good insect repellent.

Pumpkin Seed Oil

The oil from the pumpkin seeds is excellent for wounds, burns, and chapped skin. Apply directly to affected area.

Collagen Boosters

This tough, fibrous protein helps hold together cells and tissues in the body, making skin look young and smooth. Several herbs and foods have been found to boost collagen production. They are brewer's yeast, chlorella, horsetail, and thuja, particularly when horsetail and/or thuja are combined with tinctures of hawthorn, echinacea, and evening primrose oil.

Oil of Evening Primrose

Take one 500-mg. capsule a day to smooth dry, rough skin. You can also treat trouble spots by breaking open one or two capsules and applying the oil directly to the skin twice a day, after your morning shower and before bed. You can also use a body lotion that contains oil of evening primrose, especially one listing it as one of the first three ingredients. This oil also works well on atopic eczema. Take two capsules, three times a day, at least one-half hour before meals. Also apply the oil topically to affected areas.

Dandelion Root Tea

Dandelion root is excellent for troubled complexions because it cleans the liver, the body's main organ of detoxification. A toxic liver is often reflected in a spotty complexion. Drink one cup, three times a day, of the tea (using the basic decoction recipe). Or you can eat the greens as part of your salad.

Dandelion Combination Tea

This tea also works on the skin by detoxifying the liver.

Combine one ounce each of sarsaparilla root, yellow dock root, blue flag root, and dandelion root. Using one-quarter of the mixture at a time, place the herbs in one and one-half pints of boiling water and simmer for twenty to thirty minutes. Strain. Take one cup, three times a day.

Skin Healer

This traditional remedy helps to heal skin diseases such as eczema, impetigo, herpes zoster, acne, and boils.

Combine the following:

> 2 ounces of red clover blossoms
> 1 ounce of burdock root
> 1 ounce of blue flag
> ½ ounce of sassafras bark

Place one-quarter of the mixture in one pint of cold water. Bring to a boil, then simmer for twenty to thirty minutes. Cool, then strain. Take one-half cup, three times a day.

Potato Juice

This remedy for skin and scalp diseases and for overall health of the skin and hair comes from the Gypsies. Nibble on raw potato, or make a juice and drink as needed. Celery juice is also beneficial to the skin.

Honeysuckle Honey

The Gypsies mix honeysuckle with honey and light molasses to use as a healing remedy against almost all skin disorders. (They also use it as a mild laxative.)

Licorice

This herb contains antioxidant compounds which tests show lighten age spots and pigmentation caused by irritated skin when applied topically. Another active compound in licorice soothes inflammation in a way similar to hydrocortisone, but without side effects. Apply the tea (using the basic decoction recipe) to affected area and use plant-based topical skin products that list licorice among the first three ingredients.

Gingko Biloba

The oldest existing tree species known, gingkos live up to 1,000 years and their abundance of antioxidant flavenoids make them resistant to insects, disease, and pollution. Drink the tea and look for this ingredient in skin products.

Grape Seeds

The antioxidants in grape seeds are even better free radical scavengers than vitamin E and they work twice as long in the skin. Grape seeds also protect the thin walls of blood vessels from losing their strength, to prevent or correct the appearance of "spider veins." Look for skin products listing grape seed extract or oil among the first three ingredients.

Peppermint Tea Skin Toner

Made according to the basic tea recipe, the menthol in peppermint tea stimulates and cools the skin. It also possesses antiseptic properties, so it's a particularly useful skin toner.

Elderflower Wrinkle Smoother

A favorite of the English, elderflower relieves sunburn, smooths the skin, and minimizes wrinkles. Mixed with yogurt, it makes a skin-clarifying, toning, and softening mask. (Linden flower tea works in a similar manner.)

To remove freckles, place one-half cup of fresh elderflower blossoms in a container and cover with three-fourths cup of cold, distilled water. Allow to stand overnight. Strain off the liquid and use every night and morning as a wash. This also makes a good wash for bloodshot eyes.

Chamomile Oil Cleanser and Tissue Strengthener

This lotion not only cleans your skin, it strengthens delicate facial tissue, reduces swollen glands, and eases painful joints.

To prepare the oil, place three ounces of chamomile flowers in one and one-half pints of pure, cold-pressed vegetable oil. Simmer in a glass or stainless steel saucepan for forty minutes. Remove from heat and let stand overnight. Strain and bottle. Use as frequently as desired.

Gypsy Wrinkle Remover

Mix together two ounces each of white lily juice and honey with one ounce of melted white wax. Stir well before each use and apply every evening, not removing until morning.

Dry Skin Thirst Quencher

Olive oil is one of the ingredients in a time-tested remedy for dry, scaly skin. Mix two teaspoons of fine oatmeal with enough olive oil to form a soft paste. Add one-half cup of hot water and cool. Strain the mixture through muslin, squeezing thoroughly. Dab the solution on the skin two or three times a day and let it soak in. Make this preparation every other day as it will not stay fresh more than two days.

Hibiscus Astringent

A favorite in Egypt, India, and the West Indies where this flower thrives, hibiscus tea makes an excellent astringent and a stimulating bath essence.

North American Sassafras Cleanser

Whether sipped as a tea (using the basic tea recipe) or applied externally, North American sassafras cleanses and detoxifies the skin.

Rosemary Water

The water in which rosemary has been boiled contains many healing, clarifying, and soothing properties when used as a skin wash.

Rosemary Wine Wash

Boil a few handfuls of rosemary flowers in one pint of wine for fifteen minutes. Cool, bottle, and use as a face wash.

Jasmine Skin Calmer

Used as a facial steam or as a bath essence (using the basic tea recipe), this Far East delight soothes skin. When applied as a compress, it soothes tired and irritated eyes (and is said to spark libidos!).

Skin Smoothing Soak

Sea salt, when dissolved in a warm bath, calms skin and makes it silky smooth. Even ichthyosis—a thick scale usually appearing on the front of the legs—responds to a sea salt soak. Surprisingly, salt soaks make excellent moisturizers.

Brown Spot Remover

Mix one-half teaspoon of onion juice with one teaspoon of vinegar. Use as a wash as often as desired.

Brown Spot Remover II

Rub the spots with the inside of cucumber peel at least twice a day. Eventually they will bleach out.

Chapped Hands Relief

Mix together the following:

> ½ ounce of rose water
> ½ ounce of glycerin
> ¼ ounce of witch hazel extract

Mix and bottle for use. Each time you wash and dry your hands, massage this solution into your hands.

Slippery Elm Hand Wash

Brew a tea (according to the basic tea recipe) with slippery elm powder. Use as a wash for your hands as often as needed.

Blemish and Freckle Remover

Place one cup of centaury herb in two quarts of water. Add a small amount of castile soap. Leave overnight, then strain. Use as a cleansing wash.

Lemon and Rose Water Wash

Combine one ounce of powdered alum and one ounce of lemon juice. Add one pint of rose water. Bottle and shake well before using. This is also effective against freckles and blemishes.

Gypsy Freckle Wash

Dry equal amounts of wild cucumber roots and narcissus roots in a shady area. Pulverize into a fine powder. Add one-half cup of the mixture to one pint of brandy. Wash your skin with this solution until it begins to itch. Then rinse with cold water. Repeat once each day. This remedy also works on blotchy complexions.

Burdock Freckle and Blemish Wash

Make a decoction using distilled water and burdock root (using the basic decoction recipe). Cool, strain, and use morning and night as a skin wash.

Bruise Remover

Mix together equal parts of marshmallow and comfrey. Make a strong infusion (doubling the proportion of herbs to water in the basic tea recipe). Bathe affected areas frequently until the bruises disappear.

Pore Refiner

Express the juice of fresh cucumbers. Bring to boiling point. Skim the liquid and bottle it. Mix one teaspoon of the juice with two teaspoons of pure water. Apply to your face morning and night and let it dry.

Mulberry All-Purpose Mash

Pulverize a handful of mulberries in the blender at low speed, until they form a coarse mash. Use as a poultice to help heal a variety of skin conditions, including acne, ringworm, impetigo, and hives.

Acne Chaser

This tea works by helping to rid the blood of toxins that can result in acne and other skin eruptions.

Mix together the following herbs:

> 1 tablespoon sassafras
> 1 tablespoon sarsaparilla
> 1 tablespoon dandelion
> 1 tablespoon burdock
> ½ tablespoon licorice

Simmer two ounces of the herb mixture in two pints of water for thirty minutes. Drink one cup, three times a day.

Cider Vinegar Solution

Mix cider vinegar with an equal part of water to make a solution that cures impetigo and ringworm. Sponge on affected areas twice a day, and let dry.

American Indian Skin Disease Remedy

Mix together the following:

> ½ ounce sassafras bark
> 2 ounces red clover flowers
> 1 ounce burdock root
> 1 ounce blue flag root

Bring the mixture to a boil in one pint of water. Simmer for twenty minutes. Cool, then strain. Drink one-half cup three times a day, as long as the skin rash persists.

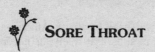 **SORE THROAT**

My Turkish grandfather always advised me to gargle with hot salt water at the first sign of a sore throat in the hope that this unpleasant practice would the kill the virus before it spread. Salt is said to loosen mucus and dry tissues, but it probably acts most effectively to draw out impurities and as an anesthetic.

Sore Throat Soother

Steep one teaspoon of crushed slippery elm bark and one-quarter teaspoon of goldenseal root in one cup of boiled water for twenty minutes. Strain and sip as needed. Do not take goldenseal for too long a period or too often; avoid it altogether if you have high blood pressure.

Sore Throat and Cough Gargle

Brew together equal parts of elder blossoms with sage leaves and tops. Make a tea approximately twice as strong as the basic tea recipe. Add honey to taste, one-quarter teaspoon of sweet almond oil and five drops of oil of clove for every one-half pint of the gargle. Gargle this mixture frequently.

Honey Herb Gargle

This also makes a great mouthwash, antiseptic and sweet-smelling.

Dissolve two tablespoons of honey in one small pint of hot sage tea (using the tea recipe). Stir in one-half pint of cider vinegar, one teaspoon sweet almond oil, and five drops of clove oil. Bottle and use as needed.

Quince

This tasty fruit was used by North American Indians to heal sore throats and mouths. Eat freely, as needed.

Persimmon

The tea made from this fruit (using the basic tea recipe) was a popular Algonquin Indian gargle for sore throats.

Black Currant Gargle

Simmer two heaping teaspoons of fresh black currants in one cup of hot water for ten minutes. Add one-half teaspoon of ground cinnamon and let the mixture stand for one-half hour. Strain and gargle while still warm. This remedy is also effective for sore gums and mouths.

Hollyhock Tea

Hollyhock leaves and flowers contain soothing properties that make it an excellent remedy for sore and irritated mouths and throats. Brew a tea (using the basic tea recipe). Take one cup, three times a day.

Horseradish Syrup

Combine grated horseradish with honey and water to make a syrup that relieves hoarse throats.

Ginger Milk Sore Throat Cure

Heat, but do not boil one pint of milk. Add two or three slices of fresh ginger or one-quarter to three-quarter teaspoons of powdered ginger, if the fresh root is not available. Simmer for ten to fifteen minutes. Serve hot with honey to taste.

Sore Throat Solution

Gargle deeply and often within the first twenty-four hours, alternating between solutions of lemon juice and very warm water, and salt and very warm water. Drink hot water mixed with lemon juice, one-quarter teaspoon of cayenne pepper, and one clove. Alternate every two hours with a drink made from hot water, apple cider vinegar, one-quarter teaspoon cayenne pepper, and one clove. Make these brews to taste—as strong as possible but not too much sweetener. Use only honey.

Fig Gargle

Chop up three to four dried figs and soak in enough water to cover overnight. Boil in one pint of water until they become pulpy. Strain and gargle with the fig water.

Sore Throat Gargle

Put one tablespoon white Karo syrup in warm water. Gargle. More soothing than gargling with salt and water and better for those watching their sodium intake.

Vinegar Gargle

Gargling with vinegar is effective any time, as the vinegar helps to maintain the proper balance of bacteria in the throat.

Vinegar-Barley Gargle

Prepare barley water by simmering one-half cup barley in one quart of water for twenty minutes. Strain. Take one cup of barley water and mix it with one teaspoon of salt and one tablespoon of cider vinegar. Stir well until salt dissolves completely. Cool and use as needed.

Herbal Gargle

Mix together the following dried herbs:

> 1 tablespoon linden leaves
> 1 tablespoon sage
> 1 tablespoon chamomile leaves and flowers
> 1 ounce oak bark

Pour one and one-half pints of boiling water over the herb mixture. Cover and steep for half an hour. Use as a gargle as needed. This also makes a great antiseptic mouthwash.

Bee Throat Cure

Gargle with juice of aloe vera (available in health food stores) and take bee propolis tablets. If you are allergic to bee pollen, just gargle with aloe vera juice twice a day.

Goldenseal and Myrrh Capsules

Combine four parts goldenseal powder with one part myrrh powder. Mix thoroughly and fill 00-size gelatin capsules. Take one or two capsules, three times day, with one-half to one cup of warm water.

Sore Throat Teas/Gargles

Take a tea made from any one or a combination of the following herbs (using the basic decoction recipe): blackberry root, slippery elm bark, ginseng root. Boil two cups of water and add one or a combination of the above and simmer for twenty minutes. With powdered herbs, use half as much.

Hot Pepper Gargle

Add one-half teaspoon of cayenne pepper to one cup of boiling water. Stir and sip while the mixture is still hot.

Echinacea/Goldenseal Tea

You can buy a tincture that combines these two herbs. Add thirty drops to a cup of warm water. Or add fifteen drops of each herb to a cup of warm water. Drink every two or three hours.

Roasted Lemon

Roast a whole lemon in your oven at 325 degrees until it breaks open. Mix one teaspoon of the juice with one-half teaspoon of honey. Drink every hour until your throat feels better.

Sage Tea

Steep a handful of fresh sage leaves in one pint of boiling water. Cover until cool. Take one-half cup, three times a day.

Sage Gargle

Combine one ounce of sage leaves with one-eighth teaspoon of cayenne powder and one pint of boiling water. Remove from heat, cover, and let it sit for twelve hours. Strain. Use for sore throats and mouth and throat ulcers as needed.

Hot Goldenseal Gargle

This tea is very effective for sore throats and gums. Add one-half tablespoon of goldenseal powder, one-half tablespoon of salt, and one-quarter tablespoon of cayenne pepper to one cup of warm water. Mix thoroughly and gargle as needed.

Pomegranate Gargle

Simmer two tablespoons of dried pomegranate rind in three cups (one and one-half pints) of water for twenty minutes or until the liquid is reduced to one pint. Strain. Gargle the juice and swallow it. This remedy is also effective against canker sores.

Fig Gargle

Add one-half ounce of finely chopped figs and one-half ounce of finely chopped marshmallow root to one pint of boiling milk. Simmer until the liquid is reduced to three-quarters of the original amount. Gargle while still warm, as needed.

Plantain Leaf Tea

Pour one cup of boiling water over one tablespoon of leaves. Steep for five to ten minutes. Swallow one tablespoon, four times a day, after meals.

Warning: If your throat does not get better in a few days, visit your doctor for a throat culture to check for a possible strep infection.

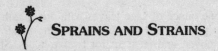

SPRAINS AND STRAINS

Horsetail Soreness Remedy

Used traditionally for pain and swelling, horsetail is especially effective in easing menstrual discomfort and speeding the healing of ankle sprains. Keep in a safe place away from children, as it can be toxic if taken internally in large quantities. Prepare according to the basic decoction recipe and apply to the affected area.

Comfrey

Comfrey contains calcium, protein, iron, and allatonin, which promote healing. Macerate the roots and leaves of this plant to make a pulp that can be placed on sprains and fractures to relieve swelling and pain. English folk call comfrey "knit-bone" and use it in setting fractures.

Myrrh, Goldenseal and Cayenne Liniment

This homemade liniment speeds healing of aching muscles, strains, soreness, sprains, swellings, and bumps. Rub into affected area, or around it if the area is too painful, three to four times a day. The liniment takes a week to make, so prepare ahead of time, before you need it.

Combine one ounce of powdered myrrh, one-half ounce of powdered goldenseal, one-quarter ounce of cayenne pepper, one pint of rubbing alcohol. Mix together and let stand seven days. Shake well daily, then pour the liquid into another bottle, leaving the sediment behind.

Hot Pepper Liniment

Boil one tablespoon of cayenne pepper in one pint of cider vinegar. Bottle the unstrained liquid while it's hot. This concoction is effective for sprains and congestion.

Arnica

Arnica tincture or ointment, which is readily available at health food stores and some pharmacies, is extremely effective when applied externally to relieve bruises, strains, sprains, sore muscles, and inflammation, and following surgery. It should be taken internally *only* in homeopathic form.

Tiger Balm

Tiger balm (oil of camphor in a petroleum base) is the Chinese equivalent of Ben Gay. It is widely available in health shops and wherever Chinese products are sold. Tiger balm is effective on sprains, as it stimulates circulation and breaks up congestion to promote speedier healing.

Willow Bark

Willow bark is a basic ingredient in aspirin and other pain killers. Soak one-half tablespoon of willow bark in two cups cold water overnight. Bring to boil and simmer for twenty minutes. Strain and cool and put in refrigerator. Sip one-quarter cup as needed.

Horse Chestnut

The ancient Turks fed this nut to their horses because of its healing properties. The nuts contain escin, a chemical used in a German- and Italian-made gel said to control the loss of water from broken blood vessels, thereby speeding healing of sprains, strains, and bruises. An ongoing international project is currently collecting and multiplying horse chestnut, selecting the nuts with the most escin and multiplying them by various propagation techniques at a research station in Edinburgh, Scotland.

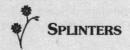

SPLINTERS

Splinter Remover

To remove a splinter under a toe or fingernail, douse the area generously with witch hazel (also an effective bruise remover) to make it easier to remove.

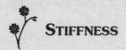

STIFFNESS

Ginger Tea

Brew a tea from the root (using the basic decoction recipe but not allowing the water to boil). Or steep one-quarter teaspoon of powdered ginger in one cup of boiling water for at least ten minutes. Drink to relieve general cramps.

Olive Oil Rub

Rub pure, cold-pressed olive oil on the soles of the feet to relieve general cramps.

Thyme Tea

Using the basic tea recipe, brew a cup of thyme tea. Take as needed to relieve general cramps.

Citrus Relaxer

Chop up one grapefruit, two oranges, and three lemons. Leave on the skins and put them in the blender. Add an equal amount of pure water and one teaspoon of cream of tartar. Drink one-quarter cup daily.

Leg Cramp Cures

Butcher's broom capsules, extracted from the root, boost circulation to the extremities and help prevent leg cramps. Take one capsule, three times a day. They can be combined with rosemary oil, which boosts circulation by strengthening capillaries.

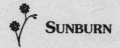

SUNBURN

Olive Oil Sunburn Soother

Mix together one-half ounce of olive oil, glycerin, and distilled witch hazel. Apply as needed for speedy relief.

Aloe Vera Gel

Apply gel from the bottle liberally or slice a leaf and place the inside on the affected area.

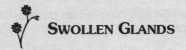

SWOLLEN GLANDS

Raspberry Juice

Drink the juice (you can buy it at your local health food store) and eat the fruit freely to combat scrofula, a tuberculous disease that swells and destroys the lymph glands. (Raspberries are also helpful in childbirth.)

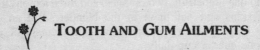

TOOTH AND GUM AILMENTS

Gum Cleanser

Combine one part goldenseal powder, one part myrrh powder, and enough water to make a paste. Wet your toothbrush and brush the teeth and the border between the gums and teeth. This antibacterial mixture is bitter but it's best if you let it stand for ten minutes. Brush teeth with this mixture three to four times a day. The bitter taste is more than compensated by the increased strength of your gums.

Sage-Myrrh Toothpaste

This concoction dates back to the nineteenth century, and it's still an excellent tooth cleanser, as well as a healing and toning treatment for your gums. Mix one tablespoon of sage powder with one ounce of powdered myrrh. Then mix together the following:

> 1 pound powdered arrow root
> 3 ounces powdered orris root
> 20 drops lemon oil
> 10 drops clove oil
> 12 drops bergamot oil

Mix all ingredients well. Moisten your toothbrush and dip into the mixture each time you brush your teeth.

Chalk–Orris Root Toothpaste

This is another excellent nineteenth-century tooth and gum treatment. Mix together the following:

> ½ ounce chalk powder
> 3 ounces orris root powder
> 4 teaspoons vanilla extract
> 15 drops rose geranium oil
> honey to achieve the desired consistency

Keep in a small, tightly covered container. Use a separate spoon or stick to scoop up desired amount and place it on your toothbrush each time you use it.

Toothache Chews

Simply chew on the leaves of the prickly ash, otherwise known as the "toothache tree." Ginger root and plantain root can be used the same way.

Strawberry Tartar Prevention

To prevent accumulation of tartar, cut a fresh, organic strawberry in half and rub the juice over your teeth. (Fresh raspberries also keep the teeth clean.)

Plantain Leaf Juice

Macerate plantain leaves to extract the juice. Swish around your mouth to combat infections of the mouth and gums.

Papaya Gum Cure

Fill your mouth with fresh papaya juice and allow it to soak. This remedy relieves sore, inflamed gums and helps to heal infections.

Grape Gum Cure

Chew grapes, including the seeds, to drain off the pus of gum infections and strengthen the tissue surrounding the teeth.

Chamomile Teething Soother

Steep one teaspoon of chamomile leaves or use ten drops of chamomile extract per one cup hot water. Cool. This tea is particularly helpful for teething infants. It can also remedy bad breath caused by an upset stomach.

Rosemary Mouthwash

Combine one-third teaspoon each of rosemary, anise, and peppermint and steep in one cup of boiling water.

Clove Toothache Relief

Always consult your dentist for any tooth and gum problems. But for relief when tooth pain strikes at a time when your dentist is unavailable, try an application of oil of cloves. The oil extracted from this common kitchen spice has numbing properties that can temporarily quiet the nerves in your tooth. Oil of cloves is available in most pharmacies and health food stores. Simply rub a cotton ball or swab soaked in the oil on the painful tooth and the immediate surrounding area. Clove oil is a well-known anesthetic, but it is very concentrated and can be irritating. Try not to get it on the gums. If you don't have the oil handy, place one or two cloves next to the affected tooth. Soak the cloves first in a small amount of hot water in a covered pot for a few minutes to activate the essential oils.

Fig Toothache Relief

Prepare a decoction using fig tree leaves (using the basic decoction recipe). Cool and drop the resulting juice into the painful tooth's cavity.

Cayenne Toothache Reliever

This versatile herb is said by some to relieve toothache pain. Clean out the tooth cavity, then saturate a small piece of absorbent cotton in cayenne pepper. Press this into the tooth cavity. It probably will burn but the relief it brings is supposed to be long-lasting.

Salt Water Tooth Pain Relief

Mix two tablespoons of salt in one cup of very hot water. Swish the mixture around your mouth to relieve toothache and cleanse the affected area. This gargle is also helpful after painful tooth and gum work.

Licorice Root

A recent study demonstrated that when glycyrrhizin, one of the active constituents of licorice, is added to toothpastes, it may help to reduce plaque buildup. Many people, especially those kicking the cigarette habit, buy the hardened root from their health food store and chew on it all day long.

Fenugreek Tea and Seeds

Simply drinking the tea and/or munching on fenugreek seeds will cause your breath and pores to exude this herb's pleasant, sweet fragrance. You could use the tea as a gargle, but why not drink it as well? Many "holistic" mouth care products, such as toothpaste and mouthwash, list fenugreek as a main ingredient.

Brew two teaspoons of seeds to one cup of boiling water. Steep for five to ten minutes, then strain.

Gum Soother

Mix one-quarter teaspoon of powdered myrrh in one-third glass of water. Rinse your mouth thoroughly. Or make a wet powder of the myrrh and apply to wet gums at night. Myrrh is also effective when mixed with an equal part of benzoin and applied to bleeding gums and gums irritated by dental work.

Juniper Berry Mouthwash

Brew a tea from juniper berries (using the basic decoction recipe). Cool, then strain. Use as a mouthwash after brushing your teeth to help heal bleeding gums.

Sage Gargle

Pour one-half pint of hot malt vinegar over one ounce of sage leaves. Add one-half pint of water. Use as a gargle for bleeding gums or for ulcers of the mouth and throat.

Lavender Flower Mouthwash

Brew a tea (using the basic tea recipe at double strength) of lavender flowers and top shoots. It not only leaves your mouth feeling refreshed and clean, but when used regularly, this mouthwash strengthens the gums.

Nettle Leaf Tea

Prepare a tea of nettle leaf (using the basic tea recipe). Cool and strain. Rinse the mouth and hold the liquid for a few moments to heal sore gums and mouth.

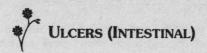

ULCERS (INTESTINAL)

Although recent research indicates that the majority of intestinal ulcers are caused by a bacterial infection, peptic ulcers result from insufficient production of hydrochloric acid, which the stomach uses to digest proteins.

Food Remedies

In the American South, okra and oatmeal are considered ulcer remedies because their demulcent properties spread a soothing coat of protection on irritated intestinal linings.

Olive Oil

This valuable food oil contains 60 percent fat and is considered a good cleansing and healing agent due to its high potassium content. Many natural healers recommend that their ulcer patients begin every meal with one teaspoon of olive oil to protect the digestive tract and exert a healing influence on intestinal ulcers.

Cabbage Juice

Freshly expressed cabbage juice, one glass taken three times daily, is said to be powerfully healing for intestinal ulcers.

Ulcer Capsules

Combine equal parts of the following herb powders: slippery elm bark, licorice, marshmallow root. Fill 00-size gelatin capsules. Take two capsules in one-half cup of warm water, three times a day, before meals.

Violet Tea

Make a tea with the dried or fresh flower (using the basic tea recipe). Drink one cup before meals, three times a day. This tea cools and soothes inflamed mucus membranes and helps to heal ulcers.

Banana Milk

Mash a banana and mix the pulp and the skin with one pint of milk. Boil for twenty minutes. Cool and drink as needed. Do not use if you are lactose intolerant.

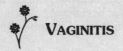

VAGINITIS

Nonspecific Vaginitis

Salt Water Baths

This is one of the most effective and gentle ways of restoring ecological balance to the vagina and eliminating nonspecific or minor infections and excess candida (yeast). Fill your bathtub with warm water. Add one-half cup of salt (sea salt is best). Sit in the tub with legs spread out for fifteen minutes and repeatedly abrade the vagina with your finger, washing out candida or any other bacteria present. Garlic is recommended by many holistic healers, but studies indicate that it is irritating to sensitive genital tissue.

Vinegar and Salt Water Douche

Alternate vinegar and salt water douches for one week. That is, douche with vinegar one day, salt water the next, etc. For the vinegar douche, mix two tablespoon of vinegar to one quart of water; for the salt douche, mix one teaspoon of salt to one quart of water. Salt neutralizes the vaginal environment. Vinegar relieves itching, but, if overused, can be drying. Use an acidophilus culture to douche the last day, made by mixing two tablespoons of acidophilus culture or organic yogurt with one pint of lukewarm water. The acidophilus restores natural bacteria and can be used once or twice a day.

Goldenseal Douche

This is effective for any vaginitis. Bring two cups of water to boil. Add one teaspoon of goldenseal powder. Simmer for twenty to thirty minutes. Let cool and strain the liquid through a cloth or pour it off the top. Add water to make one quart. Douche once a day for one week.

Goldenseal Combination Douche

Combine equal parts of goldenseal, chapparal, comfrey root, and kava kava. Make a decoction (using the basic decoction recipe). Strain, cool, and add one tablespoon of white vinegar per pint. Douche once a day, for three days.

Goldenseal Combination Capsules

Combine equal parts of goldenseal, echinacea, chapparal, and squawvine. Mix thoroughly and fill 00-size gelatin capsules. Take two capsules, three times a day, for one week only. Use in tandem with the goldenseal combination douche.

Calendula (Marigold) Douche

Bring three cups water to a boil. Remove from heat and add a handful (about four tablespoons) of calendula. Cover and let sit five to ten minutes. Cool before using. Douche once a day for one week.

Slippery Elm Douche

Douche with one ounce of powdered bark per one quart of boiled water. Steep for one hour, strain, cool, and use once a day for one week. This formula also combats genital itching.

Dandelion Tea

Place one teaspoon of the leaves, roots, or both in one cup of hot water. Steep for five minutes and strain. Drink several cups a day. This herb may also be added to salads or soups to give nourishment.

Anti-infection Implant

This implant helps clear either the vagina or anus of toxins and reduces cysts and tumors.

Mix together equal parts of the following powdered herbs: squawvine, slippery elm, yellow dock, comfrey root, marshmallow root, chickweed, goldenseal, and mullein leaves. Mix well. Add one tablespoon of the herb mixture to softened cocoa butter to make a pie dough consistency. Roll in tube form and refrigerate. Insert into the vagina at room temperature before bedtime and leave in all night.

Hollyhock Inflammation Soother

The Arabs use hollyhock tea (using the basic tea recipe) as a douche or sit bath for inflammation of the vagina and uterus. Use once a day for seven days.

Fenugreek Soothing Douche

This douche is effective in cases of vaginal irritation caused by excess mucus. Brew the tea (using the basic decoction recipe) from fenugreek seeds. Douche once a day until condition clears.

Yeast (Candida albicans and Trichomonas)

Candida and E. coli infections are caused by an overgrowth of these microorganisms, but they can be kept in check by creating a hostile environment, that is, one that favors normal desirable microorganisms. To do this, eliminate sugars and refined carbohydrates from your diet, avoid the use of antibiotics whenever possible, practice good hygiene, wear only cotton underpants, don't wear tight clothing on the lower part of your body, and eat foods like garlic and yogurt, which promote proper balance of microorganisms.

Goldenseal and Myrrh Douche

Bring three cups of water to a boil. Add one tablespoon each of goldenseal and myrrh and simmer for twenty minutes. Let the mixture sit and pour liquid off the top when it settles, or strain through a cloth. Add pure water to make one quart total. Douche once a day, for one week.

Oakstraw Tea
Make a tea (using the basic tea recipe). You can also drink the tea daily for one month along with douching no more than once a week. Make a stronger tea for the douche.

Bayberry Bark Douche
Bring one quart water to a boil. Add two or three tablespoons of bayberry bark and boil gently for twenty minutes. Strain, cool, add more water to make a quart, if necessary. Douche once a day, for one week.

Calendula or Tea Tree Oil Douche
Steep two tablespoons of calendula in a cup of boiling water for twenty minutes. Strain and cool to a comfortable temperature. Or mix four drops of tea tree oil in a cup of warm water. To use either, douche with the liquid and retain the douche for ten to fifteen minutes. Repeat twice a day, for one week.

Chickweed Douche
Boil one quart of water, and remove from the burner. Add three tablespoons of chickweed. Cover, and let sit five to ten minutes. Strain. Douche daily for one week.

Chapparal and Chamomile Douche
Take one handful each of chapparal and chamomile. Steep in one quart of boiled water for twenty minutes. Cool and strain. Douche two to three times a week for two weeks.

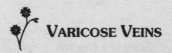

VARICOSE VEINS

Exercise your legs by walking, cycling, skipping rope, or a cross-country ski simulator. Start slowly and build up.

Cider Vinegar

Simply sponge cider vinegar on the veins to help them shrink.

White Oak Bark Tea

Brew according to basic decoction recipe. Drink one cup, three times a day, at least one-half hour before meals.

Ulcerated Veins

Apply dry powdered sugar to the veins, cover with gauze, and secure well. This will speed healing and offer antibacterial protection.

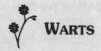

WARTS

Many of the following remedies remove warts and prevent their regrowth more effectively than removing them by burning or surgery!

Onion and Salt Dip

If you persevere, your warts will disappear after repeated applications of raw onion dipped in salt.

Garlic Poultice

Apply a poultice made of crushed garlic cloves and cover with a BandAid. Leave on for twenty-four hours. The raw garlic causes a blister to form and the warts generally fall off within a week. Apply vitamin E oil to the area to promote healing. Also effective: apply vitamin E once or twice a day or saturate the gauze portion of a gauze bandage and apply it over the wart.

Banana Cure

Apply the inside of a banana skin every day after washing the area. Tape it in place. After six weeks, the wart should disappear.

Fig Cure

Break either the leaves or branches of a fig tree. The milk that issues can be dropped on warts. Do this several times a day for two or three days. The warts should turn black and drop off.

Dandelion Cure

Squeeze the juice from the stem of a fresh dandelion. Apply three or four times a day and allow the juice to dry. The wart soon turns black and falls off. However, dandelion juice is said to be effective only when the weed is picked in the late spring or summer.

The Greater Celandine Cure

This domestic remedy works in a similar manner as dandelion stem juice. Squeeze the end of the stalk or the leaves until a drop of juice appears. Apply to the warts, three to four times a day.

Wheat Germ Oil

Apply wheat germ oil liberally to the warts, then cover with an adhesive bandage. Leave on overnight. Continue this treatment nightly for three to four weeks.

Castor Oil/Cod Liver Oil

Either of these two staples, warmed and spread on gauze and
then applied to the warts, gets rid of them in several weeks.

Thuja

Simply apply tincture of thuja on the warts with a dropper.

Appendix A:
Health-Enhancing Juices

acne: Carrot and spinach
anemia: Carrot and spinach and watercress
arthritis: Carrot and beet and cucumber *or* grapefruit
asthma: Carrot and celery *or* grapefruit
cold: Carrot and beet and cucumber *or* carrot and spinach
constipation: Carrot and spinach *or* carrot and parsley
diabetes: Carrot and celery and parsley
diarrhea: Mixed vegetables
eczema: Carrot and parsley and celery and spinach
fatigue: Carrot and spinach *or* orange and lemon and grapefruit
eyes: Carrot and celery
gout: Carrot and celery and parsley
hemorrhoids: Carrot and spinach
hypertension: Carrot and spinach and beet *or* pineapple and papaya
impotence: Carrot, parsley and cucumber *or* orange, papaya and honey
indigestion: Carrot and cabbage and beet
liver problems: Carrot and apple
peptic ulcer: Carrot and cabbage *or* pineapple and papaya

skin problems:	Carrot and cabbage *or* apple
hair problems:	Lettuce and carrot and spinach
intestinal disorders:	Papaya juice alone
vision problems:	Carrot and lettuce and parsley and spinach
for growing children:	Turnip juice (high in calcium)
for a super cleanse:	Carrot and beet and cucumber

Appendix B: Aromatherapy

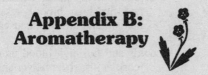

Extracted from the roots, barks, wood, leaves, flowers, or fruit of plants, these essential oils are used in massage, baths, compresses, or inhalations. The fragrances released from these essences help heal many common health problems. The following lists some of the more popular oils and the health problems they are said to help. If you apply any of the following essential oils directly to your skin, always use a carrier oil—any fine-grade, cold-pressed vegetable oil.

black pepper: colds and flu, rheumatism and arthritis, nausea

cajeput: rheumatism and arthritis

caraway: nausea

cedarwood: colds and flu

chamomile: depression, insomnia, headaches, rheumatism and arthritis, PMS

clary sage: mental fatigue, depression, high blood pressure, PMS

cypress: insomnia, varicose veins, rheumatism and arthritis, cellulite

eucalyptus: headaches, colds and flu, rheumatism and arthritis

geranium: depression, low libido, colds and flu, rheumatism and arthritis, cellulite, PMS

ginger: rheumatism and arthritis, nausea

juniper berry: mental fatigue, insomnia, high blood pressure, varicose veins, rheumatism and arthritis, cellulite

lavender: depression, insomnia, headaches, colds and flu, high blood pressure, rheumatism and arthritis, nausea, cellulite, sprains, PMS

lemon: colds and flu, high blood pressure, varicose veins, rheumatism and arthritis

mandarin orange: high blood pressure, nausea

marjoram (sweet): insomnia, headaches, high blood pressure, rheumatism and arthritis, sprains

peppermint: headaches, colds and flu, varicose veins, nausea

rosemary: mental fatigue, headaches, colds and flu, varicose veins, cellulite, sprains

sandalwood: depression, insomnia, low libido, varicose veins, nausea

tea tree: colds and flu

ylang ylang: depression, insomnia, low libido, high blood pressure

Appendix C: Recipes For Fragrant Baths

The following are some of the more popular herbs used in fragrant baths. They can also be used in essential oil form.

khus-khus: the roots of this herb are a favorite in the West Indies. They are placed in clothes drawers or closets to keep away insects and lend their delicate scent.

sandalwood: this fragrance is used as an incense in the Orient. In China, it is mixed with rice paste to make perfumed candles.

lavender: this extremely popular scent was a favorite of the Romans, who used it in their baths.

lovage: these small, yellow flowers fragrance bath water and make the bather more loveable.

roses: this crowning fragrance gives the bather the aura of a goddess.

Khus-Khus/Orris Root Bath

Combine the following:

> 10 parts borax crystals
> 4 parts cut orris roots
> 4 parts khus-khus roots
> 4 parts rose leaves
> 1 part benzoin
> 1 part sandalwood
> 1 part rose geranium

You can modify this recipe, leaving out ingredients and substituting your own.

Potpourri Bath

Mix together equal parts of bay, calamus, rosemary, chamomile, marigold flowers. Add equal parts to a quart of boiling water. Cover and simmer for ten to fifteen minutes. Strain and add to your bath water or use for a final rinse.

Mail Order Whole Foods, Supplements, Herbs, and Herbal Remedies

The Vitamin Shoppe
For catalogue, call 1-800-223-1216 M–F 8AM to 8 PM EST;
Sat–Sun 9AM to 5PM EST.
Jaffee Brothers
For catalogue, write to Valley Center, CA 92082-0636.
Clear Eye Natural Foods
For catalogue, call 1-800-724-2233.
PIA Discount Vitamins
For catalogue, call 1-800-662-8144.
Vitamin Direct
For catalogue, call 1-800-468-4027.
Vitamail Plus
For catalogue, call 1-800-964-2324.
Moonrise Herbs
For catalogue, write 1068 I Street E-W, Arcata, CA 95521 or
call 707-822-5296.
Artemis Herbs
For catalogue, write 175 Nelson Road, New Salem, MA
01364 or call 508-544-7559.
Wilderness Herbs
For catalogue, write Dept. N, Box 518, Ishpeming, MI 49849.
Women's Natural Supplements
For catalogue, call 1-800-223-3737/0394.
Hartenthaler
For catalogue, write 490 Lion Hope Road, Clayton, DE
19938.

Herbs-Liscious

For catalogue, send $2.00 to 1702 South Sixth Street, Marshalltown, IA 50158.

IMHOTEP

For catalogue, call 1-800-677-8577.

Mellengoods

For catalogue, call 1-800-649-4372.

Earthy Essentials

For catalogue, call 1-603-786-9556.

Spice Discounters

For catalogue, call 1-800-610-5950.

White Crane Trading (For herbs and seeds in bulk)

For catalogue, write 447 Tenth Avenue, New York, NY 10001.

L & H Vitamins

For catalogue, call 1-800-221-1152.

Wilner Chemists

For catalogue, call 1-800-633-1106.

The Sandy Mush Herb Nursery (For seeds and plants)

For catalogue, write 316 Surrett Cove Road, Leicester, NC 28748-9622.

Wonderful Farms (For seeds and plants)

For catalogue, call 1-800-WWHERB-1.

Pure Encapsulations (For health professionals only)

For catalogue, call 1-800-753-CAPS.

Brion Herbs (Chinese herbal formulas for health professionals only)

For catalogue, call 1-800-333-HERB.

Allergy Research Group (For health professionals only)

For catalogue, call 1-800-545-9960.

Phytompharmacy (For health professionals only)

For catalogue, call 1-800-553-2370.

Thorne Research (For health professionals only)

For catalogue, call 1-800-228-1966.

On the Internet

Ask Alice at (http://www.columbia.edu/cu/healthwise/alice.html).

Bibliography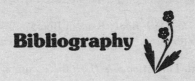

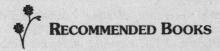 ## RECOMMENDED BOOKS

Aihara, Cornelia and Herman. *Natural Healing From Head to Toe*, Avery Publishing Group, 1994.

Balch, James F. and Phyllis A. *Prescription for Nutritional Healing*, Avery Publishing Group, 1996.

Bricklin, Mark. *Rodale's Encyclopedia of Natural Home Remedies*, Rodale Press, 1982.

Buchman, Dian Dincin. *The Complete Herbal Guide to Natural Health and Beauty*, Keats Publishing, 1995.

Colbin, Annemarie. *Food and Healing*, Ballantine Books, 1986.

Grieve, Mrs. M. *A Modern Herbal* (2 volumes), Dove, 1931; revised 1982.

Hallowell, Michael. *Herbal Healing*, Avery Publishing Group, 1994.

Hauser, Gayelord. *Treasury of Secrets*, Farrar, Straus, and Giroux, 1995.

Hill, John. *Family Herbal*, 1772.

Ismael, Richard. *The Natural Pharmacy Product Guide*, Avery Publishing Group, 1991.

Jensen, Bernard. *Nature Has a Remedy*, self-published, 1978.

Kloss, Jethro. *Back to Eden*, Woodbridge Press, 1939; revised 1981.

Lust, John. *The Herb Book*, Bantam Books, 1974.

McGarey, William A. *The Edgar Cayce Remedies*, Bantam Books, 1983.

Mindell, Earl. *Earl Mindell's Herb Bible*, Simon & Schuster, 1992.

Nambudripad, Devi. *Say Goodbye to Illness*, Delta Publishing, 1993. Order from: 6714 Beach Blvd., Buena Park, CA 90621.

Parvati, Jeannine. *Hygieia: A Woman's Herbal*, Freestone Collective, 1978.

Rector, Linda G. *Healthy Healing: An Alternative Healing Reference*, Healthy Healing Publishers, 1985.

Rodale's Illustrated Encyclopedia of Herbs, Rodale Press, 1987.

Rose, Jeanne. *Herbs & Things*, Grosset and Dunlap, 1972.

Salaman, Maureen. *Foods That Heal*, Stratford Publishing, 1989.

Tenney, Louise. *Health Handbook*, Woodland Books, 1994.

Tierra, Michael. *The Way of Herbs*, Washington Square Press, 1980.

Tisserand, Robert B. *The Art of Aromatherapy*, Destiny Books, 1977.

Valnet, Jean. *The Practice of Aromatherapy*, Destiny Books, 1980.

Weed, Susan S. *Healing Wise*, Ashtree Publishing, 1989.

Weil, Andrew. *Health and Healing*, Houghton Mifflin, 1983; revised 1988.

Weiner, Michael A. *The Herbal Bible*, Quantum Books, 1993.

Wright, Jonathan V. *Guide to Healing Nutrition*, Rodale Press, 1984.

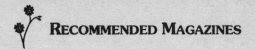

RECOMMENDED MAGAZINES

Longevity
For subscriptions call 1-800-333-2782.

New Age
For subscriptions call 1-815-734-5808 or write P.O. Box 488, Mount Morris, IL 61054-0488.

Natural Health
For subscriptions write Customer Service, P.O. Box 57320, Boulder CO 80322-7320.

Let's Live
For subscriptions call 1-800-676-4333.

The Natural Way
For subscriptions write P.O. Box 1803, Danbury, CT 06813-1803.

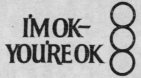

FASCINATING BOOKS
OF SPIRITUALITY
AND PSYCHIC DIVINATION

CLOUD NINE: A DREAMER'S DICTIONARY
by Sandra A. Thomson
77384-8/$6.99 US/$7.99 Can

SECRETS OF SHAMANISM:
TAPPING THE SPIRIT POWER
WITHIN YOU
by Jose Stevens, Ph.D. and Lena S. Stevens
75607-2/$5.99 US/$6.99 Can

THE LOVERS' TAROT
by Robert Mueller, Ph.D., and Signe E. Echols, M.S.,
with Sandra A. Thomson
76886-0/$11.00 US/$13.00 Can

SEXUAL ASTROLOGY
by Marlene Masini Rathgeb
76888-7/$11.00 US/$15.00 Can

SPIRITUAL TAROT: SEVENTY-EIGHT
PATHS TO PERSONAL DEVELOPMENT
by Signe E. Echols, M.S., Robert Mueller, Ph.D.,
and Sandra A. Thomson
78206-5/$12.00 US/$16.00 Can

THE NATIONWIDE #1 BESTSELLER

the Relaxation Response

by Herbert Benson, M.D.
with Miriam Z. Klipper

A SIMPLE MEDITATIVE TECHNIQUE
THAT HAS HELPED MILLIONS
TO COPE WITH
FATIGUE, ANXIETY AND STRESS

Available Now—
00676-6/ $6.99 US/ $8.99 Can